Child Abuse and Neglect: Advancements and Challenges in the 21st Century

Guest Editor

ANDREW SIROTNAK, MD

PEDIATRIC CLINICS
OF NORTH AMERICA

www.pediatric.theclinics.com

April 2009 • Volume 56 • Number 2

SAUNDERS an imprint of ELSEVIER, Inc.

W.B. SAUNDERS COMPANY
A Division of Elsevier Inc.

1600 John F. Kennedy Boulevard ● Suite 1800 ● Philadelphia, Pennsylvania 19103-2899

http://www.theclinics.com

THE PEDIATRIC CLINICS OF NORTH AMERICA Volume 56, Number 2
April 2009 ISSN 0031-3955, ISBN-13: 978-1-4377-0519-5, ISBN-10: 1-4377-0519-7

Editor: Carla Holloway
Developmental Editor: Theresa Collier

The Pediatric Clinics of North America (ISSN 0031-3955) is published bimonthly by Elsevier Inc., 360 Park Avenue South, New York, NY 10010-1710. Months of publication are February, April, June, August, October, and December. Business and Editorial Offices: 1600 John F. Kennedy Blvd., Suite 1800, Philadelphia, PA 19103-2899. Customer Service Office: 11830 Westline Industrial Drive, St. Louis, MO 63146. Periodicals postage paid at New York, NY and additional mailing offices. Subscription prices are $162.00 per year (US individuals), $350.00 per year (US institutions), $220.00 per year (Canadian individuals), $466.00 per year (Canadian institutions), $262.00 per year (international individuals), $466.00 per year (international institutions), $81.00 per year (US students and residents), and $138.00 per year (international and Canadian residents and students). To receive students/resident rare, orders must be accompanied by name of affiliated institution, date of term, and the signature of program/residency coordinator on institution letterhead. Orders will be billed at individual rate until proof of status is received. Foreign air speed delivery is included in all *Clinics* subscription prices. All prices are subject to change without notice. **POSTMASTER:** Send address changes to *The Pediatric Clinics of North America*, Elsevier Journals Customer Service, 11830 Westline Industrial Drive, St. Louis, MO 63146. **Customer Service: 1-800-654-2452 (US and Canada). From outside of the US and Canada: 1-314-453-7041. Fax: 1-314-453-5170. For print support, e-mail: JournalsCustomerService-usa@elsevier.com. For online support, e-mail: JournalsOnlineSupport-usa@elsevier.com.**

Reprints. For copies of 100 or more, of articles in this publication, please contact the Commercial Reprints Department, Elsevier Inc., 360 Park Avenue South, New York, NY 10010-1710. Tel.: 212-633-3812; Fax: 212-462-1935; E-mail: reprints@elsevier.com.

The Pediatric Clinics of North America is also published in Spanish by McGraw-Hill Inter-americana Editores S.A., Mexico City, Mexico; in Portuguese by Riechmann and Affonso Editores, Rua Comandante Coelho 1085, CEP 21250, Rio de Janeiro, Brazil; and in Greek by Althayia SA, Athens, Greece.

The Pediatric Clinics of North America is covered in *MEDLINE/PubMed (Index Medicus), Excerpta Medica, Current Contents, Current Contents/Clinical Medicine, Science Citation Index, ASCA, ISI/BIOMED,* and *BIOSIS.*

Printed and bound by CPI Group (UK) Ltd, Croydon, CR0 4YY

Transferred to Digital Print 2011

GOAL STATEMENT
The goal of the *Pediatric Clinics of North America* is to keep practicing physicians and residents up to date with current clinical practice in pediatrics by providing timely articles reviewing the state-of-the-art in patient care.

ACCREDITATION
The *Pediatric Clinics of North America* is planned and implemented in accordance with the Essential Areas and Policies of the Accreditation Council for Continuing Medical Education (ACCME) through the joint sponsorship of the University of Virginia School of Medicine and Elsevier. The University of Virginia School of Medicine is accredited by the ACCME to provide continuing medical education for physicians.

The University of Virginia School of Medicine designates this educational activity for a maximum of 15 *AMA PRA Category 1 Credits*™. Physicians should only claim credit commensurate with the extent of their participation in the activity.

The American Medical Association has determined that physicians not licensed in the US who participate in this CME activity are eligible for 15 *AMA PRA Category 1 Credits*™.

Credit can be earned by reading the text material, taking the CME examination online at http://www.theclinics.com/home/cme, and completing the evaluation. After taking the test, you will be required to review any and all incorrect answers. Following completion of the test and evaluation, your credit will be awarded and you may print your certificate.

FACULTY DISCLOSURE/CONFLICT OF INTEREST
The University of Virginia School of Medicine, as an ACCME accredited provider, endorses and strives to comply with the Accreditation Council for Continuing Medical Education (ACCME) Standards of Commercial Support, Commonwealth of Virginia statutes, University of Virginia policies and procedures, and associated federal and private regulations and guidelines on the need for disclosure and monitoring of proprietary and financial interests that may affect the scientific integrity and balance of content delivered in continuing medical education activities under our auspices.

The University of Virginia School of Medicine requires that all CME activities accredited through this institution be developed independently and be scientifically rigorous, balanced and objective in the presentation/discussion of its content, theories and practices.

All authors/editors participating in an accredited CME activity are expected to disclose to the readers relevant financial relationships with commercial entities occurring within the past 12 months (such as grants or research support, employee, consultant, stock holder, member of speakers bureau, etc.). The University of Virginia School of Medicine will employ appropriate mechanisms to resolve potential conflicts of interest to maintain the standards of fair and balanced education to the reader. Questions about specific strategies can be directed to the Office of Continuing Medical Education, University of Virginia School of Medicine, Charlottesville, Virginia.

The faculty and staff of the University of Virginia Office of Continuing Medical Education have no financial affiliations to disclose.

The authors/editors listed below have identified no financial or professional relationships for themselves or their spouse/partner:
Randell Alexander, MD, PhD; Donald C. Bross, JD, PhD; Antonia Chiesa, MD; Nancy Donelan-McCall, PhD; Howard Dubowitz, MD, MS; Ann-Christine Duhaime, MD; Michael Durfee, MD: John Eckenrode, PhD; Carla Holloway (Acquisitions Editor); Richard D. Krugman, MD; Alex V. Levin, MD, MHSc; Robin Mekonnen, MSW; Kathleen G. Noonan, JD; Juan M. Parra, MD, MPH; Karen Rheuban, MD (Test Author); David Rubin, MD, MSCE; Kimberly Shipman, PhD; Andrew Sirotnak, MD (Guest Editor); Heather Taussig, PhD; and Kathryn Wells, MD, FAAP.

The authors/editors listed below identified the following professional or financial affiliations for themselves or their spouse/partner:
David L. Olds, PhD has a contract to conduct research for Nurse Family Partnership.

Disclosure of Discussion of Non-FDA Approved Uses for Pharmaceutical and/or Medical Devices:
The University of Virginia School of Medicine, as an ACCME provider, requires that all authors identify and disclose any "off label" uses for pharmaceutical and medical device products. The University of Virginia School of Medicine recommends that each physician fully review all the available data on new products or procedures prior to clinical use.

TO ENROLL
To enroll in the *Pediatric Clinics of North America* Continuing Medical Education program, call customer service at 1-800-654-2452 or visit us online at www.theclinics.com/home/cme. The CME program is available to subscribers for an additional fee of $195.00.

Contributors

GUEST EDITOR

ANDREW SIROTNAK, MD
Associate Professor of Pediatrics, University of Colorado School of Medicine; and
Director, Kempe Child Protection Team, The Children's Hospital, Aurora, Colorado

AUTHORS

RANDELL ALEXANDER, MD, PhD
Professor of Pediatrics and Chief, Division of Child Protection and Forensic Pediatrics,
University of Florida–Jacksonville, Jacksonville, Florida

DONALD C. BROSS, JD, PhD
Professor, The Kempe Center for the Prevention and Treatment of Child Abuse
and Neglect, University of Colorado School of Medicine, Aurora, Colorado

ANTONIA CHIESA, MD
Senior Instructor, University of Colorado School of Medicine, Department of Pediatrics;
and Kempe Child Protection Team, The Children's Hospital, Aurora, Colorado

NANCY DONELAN-McCALL, PhD
Assistant Professor, Department of Pediatrics, University of Colorado Denver, Aurora,
Colorado

HOWARD DUBOWITZ, MD, MS
Professor of Pediatrics, Department of Pediatrics, University of Maryland School of
Medicine; Director, Center for Families, University of Maryland; and Chief, Division of Child
Protection, Department of Pediatrics, University of Maryland Hospital, Baltimore,
Maryland

ANN-CHRISTINE DUHAIME, MD
Associate Professor, Department of Pediatric Neurosurgery, Children's Hospital
at Dartmouth, Dartmouth Hitchcock Medical Center, Hanover, New Hampshire

MICHAEL DURFEE, MD
Department of Pediatrics, Division of General Pediatrics, University of Texas Health
Science Center at San Antonio Medical School, San Antonio, Texas

JOHN ECKENRODE, PhD
Professor, Department of Human Development, College of Human Ecology; and Director
of Family Life Development Center, Cornell University, Ithaca, New York

RICHARD D. KRUGMAN, MD
Vice Chancellor for Health Affairs and Dean, University of Colorado School of Medicine,
Denver, Colorado

ALEX V. LEVIN, MD, MHSc
Chief, Pediatric Ophthalmology and Ocular Genetics, Wills Eye Institute, Philadelphia, Pennsylvania

ROBIN MEKONNEN, MSW
PolicyLab: Center to Bridge Research, Practice, and Policy at The Children's Hospital of Philadelphia; and School of Social Policy and Practice, The University of Pennsylvania, Philadelphia, Pennsylvania

KATHLEEN NOONAN, JD
Managing Director, PolicyLab: Center to Bridge Research, Practice, and Policy at The Children's Hospital of Philadelphia, Philadelphia, Pennsylvania

DAVID L. OLDS, PhD
Professor, Department of Pediatrics; Department of Psychiatry; Department of Nursing; Department of Preventative Medicine; and Director, Prevention Research Center for Family and Child Health, University of Colorado Denver, Aurora, Colorado

JUAN M. PARRA, MD, MPH
Associate Professor and Interim Division Head of General Pediatrics, University of Texas Health Science Center at San Antonio Medical School, San Antonio, Texas

DAVID RUBIN, MD, MSCE
PolicyLab: Center to Bridge Research, Practice, and Policy at The Children's Hospital of Philadelphia; and Department of Pediatrics, University of Pennsylvania School of Medicine, Philadelphia, Pennsylvania

KIMBERLY SHIPMAN, PhD
Assistant Professor, University of Colorado School of Medicine, The Kempe Center for the Prevention and Treatment of Child Abuse and Neglect, Aurora, Colorado

HEATHER TAUSSIG, PhD
Associate Professor, University of Colorado School of Medicine, The Kempe Center for the Prevention and Treatment of Child Abuse and Neglect, Aurora, Colorado

KATHRYN WELLS, MD, FAAP
Community Pediatrician, Community Health Services, Denver Health; Medical Director, Denver Family Crisis Center, Denver; Assistant Professor of Pediatrics, Department of Pediatrics, University of Colorado School of Medicine, Aurora, Colorado

Contents

Preface xi

Andrew Sirotnak

Abusive Head Trauma 317

Antonia Chiesa and Ann-Christine Dunhaime

Child physical abuse that results in injury to the head or brain has been described using many terms, including battered child syndrome, whiplash injuries, shaken infant or shaken impact syndrome, and nonmechanistic terms such as abusive head trauma or nonaccidental trauma. These injuries sustained by child abuse victims are discussed in detail in this article, including information about diagnosis, management and outcomes. The use of forensics, the use imaging studies, and associated injuries are also detailed.

Retinal Hemorrhages: Advances in Understanding 333

Alex V. Levin

Retinal hemorrhage is a cardinal manifestation of abusive head injury characterized by repetitive acceleration-deceleration with or without blunt head impact. Detailed description of the hemorrhages and documentation are critical to diagnosis. Vitreoretinal traction appears to be the major causative factor. Outcome is largely dependent on brain and optic nerve injury.

Substance Abuse and Child Maltreatment 345

Kathryn Wells

Pediatricians and other medical providers caring for children need to be aware of the dynamics in the significant relationship between substance abuse and child maltreatment. A caregiver's use and abuse of alcohol, marijuana, heroin, cocaine, methamphetamine, and other drugs place the child at risk in multiple ways. Members of the medical community need to understand these risks because the medical community plays a unique and important role in identifying and caring for these children. Substance abuse includes the abuse of legal drugs as well as the use of illegal drugs. The abuse of legal substances may be just as detrimental to parental functioning as abuse of illicit substances. Many substance abusers are also polysubstance users and the compounded effect of the abuse of multiple substances may be difficult to measure. Often other interrelated social features, such as untreated mental illness, trauma history, and domestic violence, affect these families.

Tackling Child Neglect: A Role for Pediatricians 363

Howard Dubowitz

Child neglect, the most prevalent form of maltreatment, poses challenges for pediatricians. There often is uncertainty regarding what constitutes neglect and how best to address it. The complexity is compounded by the many ways neglect can manifest. This article first discusses why neglect is so important a concern and then provides definitional considerations and a description of forms of neglect. Next presented are principles for assessing and addressing neglect and suggestions for prevention and advocacy.

Child Fatality Review Teams   379

Michael Durfee, Juan M. Parra, and Randell Alexander

The history of child fatality review (CFR) begins with the work of Ambrose Tardieu in 1860. More than a century later, in 1978, the first team was established in Los Angeles, California. This article reviews the history of CFR, the composition of teams, and its purpose based in preventive public health. The successes of three decades and challenges for the future of CFR are discussed.

Home Visiting for the Prevention of Child Maltreatment: Lessons Learned During the Past 20 Years   389

Nancy Donelan-McCall, John Eckenrode, and David L. Olds

For nearly two decades, home visitation has been promoted as a promising strategy to prevent child maltreatment, but reviews of the literature on home visiting programs have been mixed. This article examines how home visitation for the prevention of child maltreatment has evolved during the past 20 years. It reviews several home visitation programs focused on preventing child maltreatment and highlights the Nurse-Family Partnership home visitation program. It discusses how advocacy and public policy for prevention of child maltreatment have shifted from a general call to promote universal home visitation programs to a more refined emphasis on promoting programs that are evidence-based, targeted to those most at risk for maltreatment, and with infrastructure in place to ensure implementation with fidelity to the model tested in trials. Finally, it discusses how primary care providers may advocate to ensure that their patients have access to evidence-based home visiting programs that meet their needs.

Achieving Better Health Care Outcomes for Children in Foster Care   405

Robin Mekonnen, Kathleen Noonan, and David Rubin

This article reviews the challenges health care systems face as they attempt to improve health care outcomes for children in foster care. It discusses several of the promising health care strategies occurring outside the perimeter of child welfare and identifies some of the key impasses in working alongside efforts in child welfare reform. The authors posit that the greatest impasse in establishing a reasonable quality of health care for these children is placement instability, in which children move frequently among multiple homes and in and out of the child welfare system. The authors propose potential strategies in which efforts to improve placement stability can serve as a vehicle for multidisciplinary reform across the health care system.

**Mental Health Treatment of Child Abuse and Neglect: The Promise
of Evidence-Based Practice**   417

Kimberly Shipman and Heather Taussig

In 2006, 3.6 million children in the United States received a child protective services' investigation and 905,000 children (about one-quarter of those investigated) were found to have been abused or neglected. Children who have been maltreated are at risk for experiencing a host of mental health problems, including depression, posttraumatic stress, dissociation, reactive attachment, low self-esteem, social problems, suicidal behavior, aggression, conduct disorder, attention-deficit hyperactivity disorder (ADHD) and problem behaviors, including delinquency, risky sexual behavior and substance use. Given the high rate of mental health problems, it is not surprising that maltreated youth are in need of mental health services. Unfortunately, only a fraction of these children and adolescents receive services. Recently, several evidence-based practices have been rigorously tested and are demonstrating efficacy in reducing mental health problems associated with maltreatment. This article details these developments.

Child Maltreatment Law and Policy as a Foundation for Child Advocacy   429

Donald C. Bross and Richard D. Krugman

Advocacy for children is a fundamental pediatric concern and activity. Notwithstanding achievements for children to date, pediatrics can do more in the twenty-first century to advocate for children and promote research on ways in which advocacy for children can be improved. Evidence-based advocacy should take many directions including legislation, system change in local and state agencies such as social services and health departments, financial assistance including Medicaid, evidence provided to courts at trial and on appeal through "friend of the court" participation, family guidance, public education, and the promotion of pediatric law and bioethics.

Index   441

FORTHCOMING ISSUES

June 2009
Advances in Neonatology
Lucky Jain, MD, and David Carlton, MD,
Guest Editors

August 2009
Pediatric Quality
Leonard Feld, MD, and Shabnam Jain, MD,
Guest Editors

October 2009
Nutritional Deficiencies
Praveen S. Goday, MD, and
Timothy Sentongo, MD, *Guest Editors*

RECENT ISSUES

February 2009
**Common Respiratory Symptoms and
Illnesses: A Graded Evidence-Based Approach**
Anne B. Chang, MBBS, MPHTM, FRACP, PhD,
Guest Editor

December 2008
Developmental Disabilities, Part II
Donald E. Greydanus, MD,
Dilip R. Patel, MD, and
Helen D. Pratt, PhD, *Guest Editors*

October 2008
Developmental Disabilities, Part I
Donald E. Greydanus, MD,
Dilip R. Patel, MD, and
Helen D. Pratt, PhD, *Guest Editors*

RELATED INTEREST

Pediatric Clinics of North America
February 2006 (Volume 53, Issue 1)
Pediatric Emergencies, Part I
Donald Van Wie, Ghazala Q. Sharieff, and James E. Colletti, *Guest Editors*
www.pediatric.theclinics.com

THE CLINICS ARE NOW AVAILABLE ONLINE!

Access your subscription at:
www.theclinics.com

Preface

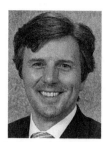

Andrew Sirotnak, MD
Guest Editor

This issue of *Pediatric Clinics of North America* focusing on child abuse and neglect follows an issue that was produced nearly 20 years ago, in 1991. Now, 50 years after the establishment of the first hospital-based, multidisciplinary child protection teams, this collection of articles looks at the challenges for the current century. There is always the need for ongoing education in this area of pediatrics. Battered children still die from severe injuries, sexually abused children may be victimized repeatedly, the number of children who have overwhelming needs in foster care has increased, and their stressed, burdened families often have limited or no access to medical care and mental health treatment. Existing resources may be managed by child welfare and health care systems that, while populated with dedicated and caring professionals, are pushed to their own limits of operational functionality and financial crisis. Effective advocacy for these children must flow from our up-to-date knowledge and clinical practice.

There have been great clinical advancements in the field and a notable increase in the body of peer-reviewed literature. This progress has paralleled the realization that the quality of our work must be supported by a strong evidence base and markers of effective outcomes. This approach in medicine is not new, and, indeed, clinicians in private, academic, and hospital-based pediatrics have, in the past decade, embraced this manner of practice—or had it forced upon them—with the ultimate goal of providing care that is best for children and families. In the area of child abuse, this is a challenging and often difficult approach, given the unique circumstances of child abuse cases. The ability to perform clinical studies may be hampered, for example, by the inherent inconsistent histories provided in child abuse cases or by the need to protect the confidentiality of child welfare information or other investigation data. Despite these challenges, we have a growing body of literature reflecting quality research into the incidence, epidemiology, spectrum of injuries, and outcomes of all forms of child maltreatment. Randomized controlled trials in this field have also provided us important data on the prevention and treatment of child abuse.

In this issue, Chiesa and Duhaime review what is known and what we are learning about abusive head trauma, our most preventable form of physical abuse. Clinical experience, new imaging modalities, court challenges to our science, and basic research have all added to our growing knowledge base. International ophthalmologist expert Alex Levin updates us on the current knowledge and evidence base on retinal hemorrhages.

Pediatr Clin N Am 56 (2009) xi–xii
doi:10.1016/j.pcl.2009.03.008
0031-3955/09/$ – see front matter
pediatric.theclinics.com

He reviews the advances in the understanding of mechanism, animal-model research, exam documentation, and outcomes of this finding in abusive head trauma.

Wells presents a thorough review of the state of the literature and practice related to substance abuse and child maltreatment, with a focus on the national crisis of methamphetamine abuse. Her article on this longstanding and growing problem is a nonjudgmental call for increased attention to this issue affecting many families. Dubowitz reviews the complexity of defining, assessing, and preventing child neglect in a very thoughtful article for the reader. His general principles are a helpful template for the primary care clinician. Durfee, Parra, and Alexander review the three decades history of Child Fatality Review Teams and the successful public health impact of these multidisciplinary programs.

Prevention of child abuse and neglect has received much national attention from a federal funding perspective. Olds and colleagues review their nearly three decades of research on prevention, the related medical literature, and present a detailed analysis of home-visitation models. More than any other area in this field, there is hope for continued success with the rigorously tested interventions for at-risk families. Likewise, Shipman and Taussig present a fine review of evidenced-based practice treatment models for maltreated children. While describing specific programs and projects, their article also brings sharp focus to the concept of evidence-based practice for the general clinician reader and how this practice can be applied to the treatment of abused children.

In a thought provoking article on the state of health care for children in foster and out-of-home care, Mekonnen and colleagues challenge us to revise our approach to improving health care outcomes for these children. The collaborative spirit of a coordinated, interdisciplinary approach for which they advocate is rooted in the history of this field and promises to change its very future. Finally, Bross and Krugman close our issue with an article that reframes the concept of pediatric advocacy. Starting with a brief retrospective of Kempe, his colleagues, and those that followed, they recommend to us an evidence-based approach to policy that is supported by research, stories of success, and true career development, especially in pediatric law and bioethics, for our current generation of pediatric leaders.

Pediatricians and all primary care providers continue to be the leaders in this field. Child Abuse Pediatrics was recognized as an American Board of Pediatrics subspecialty area, with program accreditation and certifying exams to come soon. The American Academy of Pediatrics continues to advocate for these children within its active section of Child Abuse and Neglect. Senior faculty, mentors, and researchers in the fields of general pediatrics, child abuse, mental health, health care outcomes, and child welfare policy are engaged as never before in the training and mentoring of new clinician leaders and researchers. Through continued collaborative work, reaching out to colleagues in the areas of genetics, biomechanics, neurobiology, and others, child abuse pediatrics, with a half century as a strong base, is poised to develop further as a vibrant field. Our focus will always remain on compassionate care, quality outcomes, and unwavering advocacy for all maltreated children and their families.

Andrew Sirotnak, MD
Child Abuse and Neglect
The Children's Hospital
13123 East 16th Avenue, B-138
Aurora, CO 80045, USA

E-mail address:
Sirotnak.Andrew@tchden.org

Abusive Head Trauma

Antonia Chiesa, MD[a],*, Ann-Christine Duhaime, MD[b]

KEYWORDS

- Child abuse • Abusive head trauma
- Pediatric traumatic brain injury • Shaken baby syndrome
- Nonaccidental trauma

Child physical abuse that results in injury to the head or brain has been described using many terms, which have evolved over the past half-century or more. These items have included the battered child syndrome, whiplash injuries, shaken infant or shaking impact syndrome, and nonmechanistic terms such as abusive head trauma or nonaccidental trauma.[1–7] This evolution has occurred as the spectrum of injuries—and the mechanisms that are potentially responsible for them—have been studied in increasing detail in multiple clinical series from around the world, as well as with pathophysiologic and biomechanical modeling. Because children may present with varying histories, physical findings, and radiologic findings, the terms "inflicted head injury," "nonaccidental trauma," and "abusive head trauma" are used in this article to reflect those constellations of injuries that are caused by the directed application of force to an infant or young child resulting in physical injury to the head and/or its contents. These injuries most often include subdural and/or subarachnoid hemorrhage, with varying degrees of neurologic signs and symptoms. A high proportion of children also present with retinal hemorrhages, physical or radiologic evidence of contact to the head, upper cervical spine injuries, and skeletal injuries. These features are described in more detail in the following section.

Use of the more general terms reflects an attempt to avoid the pitfalls of assuming the exact mechanism of injury; the general terms also encompass a wide range of traumatic forces, which are potentially harmful and can result in different patterns of neurotrauma. These forces include: blunt force trauma, acceleration/deceleration (inertial) forces, penetrating trauma, and asphyxiation.

EPIDEMIOLOGY

Establishing incidence data for abusive head trauma has been challenging, in part because of the definitional issues noted; however, several studies have attempted to examine issues of epidemiology. Early studies revealed that inflicted injuries

[a] Department of Pediatrics, Kempe Child Protection Team, The Children's Hospital, 13123 E. 16th Avenue, Box 138, Denver, CO 80045, USA
[b] Department of Pediatric Neurosurgery, Children's Hospital at Dartmouth, Dartmouth Hitchcock Medical Center, One Medical Center Drive, Lebanon, NH 03756, USA
* Corresponding author.
E-mail address: Chiesa.Antonia@tchden.org (A. Chiesa).

Pediatr Clin N Am 56 (2009) 317–331
doi:10.1016/j.pcl.2009.02.001
0031-3955/09/$ – see front matter © 2009 Elsevier Inc. All rights reserved.

make up a significant portion of traumatic brain injury in children younger than 2 years of age, and such injuries account for serious morbidity and mortality in that group.[8,9] When compared with accidental head injury, the hospital length-of-stay and medical costs incurred from abusive head trauma are higher.[10]

A recent study out of North Carolina found an incidence of inflicted brain injury in the first two years of life of 17.0 per 100,000 person-years.[11] Another prospective study from Scotland during 1998–1999 found an annual incidence of 24.6 per 100,000 children younger than 1 year (a higher rate than a previous 15-year retrospective study done in the same county).[12] The authors of that study suggested that the discrepancies between the prospective and retrospective study outcomes reflect the challenge of tracking the problem caused by lack of a single international classification of diseases (ICD) code to describe the medical findings.

This challenge and others were addressed at a 2008 symposium and later summarized in articles to a supplement to the *Journal of Preventative Medicine*. The symposium was convened, in part, to discuss definitional issues regarding inflicted brain injury, as well as methods for measuring its incidence. In his commentary, Alexander Butchart, PhD, argues that determining the epidemiology of child maltreatment will help elucidate the issue as a public health concern and lead to the formation of larger scale prevention efforts.[13]

MECHANISMS

In 1946, Dr. John Caffey first recognized a possible traumatic association between head injuries and fractures in infants.[14] In the following three decades, important work by Silverman,[15] Ommaya,[16] and Guthkelch,[3] contributed to the acknowledgment of child abuse as a medical condition. Noting that many of his patients presented without a clear mechanism of trauma to explain their injuries, in 1974, Caffey coined the term "the whiplash shaken infant syndrome."[4] He used the term to describe the constellation of injuries that includes subdural hematoma, long bone fractures, and retinal hemorrhages; these are symptoms that, in the absence of a reasonable history of trauma or other medical condition, are still considered hallmarks for abusive head injury. The idea that shaking might be causative was first proposed by Norman Guthkelch, a neurosurgeon who, working with pediatricians and social workers, obtained some histories of violent shaking as a part of the injury scenario.[3] In contrast, Caffey's initial concept was that shaking might be injurious even when performed by well-meaning caretakers as a generally accepted form of discipline, because of the presumed inherent fragility of young infants.[17] These authors were aware of experiments in primates, whose heads were subjected to large magnitude angular decelerations involving crashes in high-velocity sleds, leading to unconsciousness and subdural hemorrhage.[18] Thus, the idea of angular deceleration as the causative mechanism for subdural hematoma was hypothesized as the necessary mechanism in infant shaking injuries.

Over the ensuing decades, other authors noted a high incidence of contact injuries, including scalp hematomas, skull fractures, and brain contusions, in abused infants; the injuries were visible either clinically, radiologically, or at autopsy.[19–21] Biomechanical models of young infants were developed that suggested that even violent manual shaking caused angular decelerations that were very low compared with those required to cause concussive or hemorrhagic injury in primates, but that inflicted impacts were associated with angular decelerations that were approximately 50 times greater and within the range thought more likely to be associated with brain injury.[19,22] It was suggested that physical evidence of impact might not be seen if the deformable infant head stopped suddenly against a relatively soft surface, but large magnitude angular deceleration would still occur from this type of impact. Other authors created alternative physical models that suggested that shaking alone might generate sufficient force to be injurious.[23] Additionally, the frequent finding of upper cervical or cervicomedullary injury became increasingly recognized, although the mechanisms required to cause this type of injury and the exact contribution to the clinical constellation remains incompletely understood. Almost all infants with inflicted injuries who are found at autopsy to have cervical spine injuries also have subdural hemorrhage and other typical findings, which seem unlikely to be related only to spinal injury.[24–26]

Finally, the contributions of the initial history to the understanding of mechanism, as well as confessions by admitted perpetrators, have suggested that various scenarios may occur in the setting of violent inflicted injury in infants and young children. Although some caretakers mention shaking, this history is given spontaneously in the minority of cases in most series.[14,21,27] A history of a short-height fall or no history of trauma (that is, the child presents because of symptoms) are the most common initial histories given.[28] Although some confessions mention shaking, others involve throwing, striking, or other violent mechanisms. For all these reasons, terminology that does not suggest a specific mechanism of injury has become preferred by most professional organizations. Position papers published by such entities as the American Academy of Pediatrics[29] and the National Association of Medical Examiners[30] reflect the evolution of the medical literature over a relatively short period of time.

DIAGNOSIS

Determining whether a child's injuries are the result of child physical abuse can be a difficult process. If a traumatic cause is not readily apparent, careful assessment is warranted. Glick and Staley propose that a detailed evaluation by a multidisciplinary child protection team has become standard of care in many facilities.[31] Teams are typically directed by a child abuse trained pediatrician (subspecialty board certification available in 2009) and may include members from other medical and surgical disciplines, as well as medical social work. This approach ensures a thorough consideration of all the factors involved, including the medical and social issues, so that a final diagnosis is reached objectively.

A core component of the diagnostic process is a comprehensive history of presenting illness. The initial history should include details about timeline of symptoms and the exact events leading up to the present, including a detailed description of the events before and after the child became symptomatic. When there is a history of trauma, a detailed description of exactly what happened, what position the child was in, how the child landed, what the fall height was, how the child acted immediately afterwards and thereafter, and what the caretakers did is invaluable in reconstructing the injury events.[8] Included in this history should be: who has cared for the child; the relationship between caretakers and the child; birth/past medical history; prior trauma; and family history, particularly any history of bleeding disorders. Care should be taken not to lead the history by suggesting whether specific mechanisms or actions might have occurred; it is preferable to simply ask open-ended questions and to seek specific answers, such as: "What happened next?" or "What did you do then?" or "What did he/she look like/do?"

Focusing the history on the identification of a trigger for abuse by the caretaker may also be helpful. A commonly described trigger is crying. Abusive head trauma incidence curves correlate with periods of normal crying,[32] colic, and immunizations. Other triggers in older children include temperament, behavior, and toileting.

Obviously, the psychosocial stressors may affect a caregiver's coping skills and contribute to poor parenting or the potential for impulse control issues. After stabilization of the child, additional details can be ascertained by a multidisciplinary assessment by the medical providers, child protection personnel, and a social work team. A full psychosocial history will screen for preexisting mental health diagnoses, prior concerns of child maltreatment, and other risk factors, such as substance abuse or domestic violence.

As previously stated, abusive head injury is well recognized as a common cause of brain injury in children younger than 2 years of age, with the majority of such injuries being in the first year of life.[8,9] It also should be noted that case reports have documented its occurrence in older children.[33] In a prospective study of 66 children 36-months-old or younger with subdural hematoma, Feldman and colleagues found that 59% of the patients sustained their injury from abuse. Those patients were more likely than the accidentally injured children to have retinal hemorrhage and fractures. An important distinguishing feature was that the abused patients presented with no history of trauma or a history of a minor fall. All the accidental injuries occurred from a motor vehicle accident or a clearly documented major trauma.[34] Absent, inconsistent (eg, developmentally or mechanistically implausible) or evolving histories to explain a traumatic injury in a child can be a red flag for child physical abuse.

Although it is commonly accepted that abuse occurs across all socioeconomic demographics, there may be demographic differences in families of patients with abusive head injury as compared with the general population. Specifically victims and perpetrators are more commonly male. Parents of the patients are more likely to be young, unmarried, less educated, or from a minority group; mothers are more likely to smoke during the pregnancy, have late prenatal care, and to have delivered a low birth weight child.[35] Some point out that the outcomes may correlate with poverty status or reflect a bias in reporting for concerns of abusive head trauma.[35] More research will help clarify the issue; however, studies such as this illustrate the importance of including a social history with the medical evaluation.

Analysis of perpetrators' confession data also reflects a predominance of male perpetrators; Starling and colleagues[36] found that perpetrators are most likely to be fathers, followed by boyfriends, female babysitters, and mothers, in descending order. Some confessions have supported the notion that children are immediately symptomatic after serious trauma is inflicted. Perpetrators are more likely to confess if the victim is younger or impaired at hospital discharge.[37]

The spectrum of brain pathology observed from abusive head injury varies. Abnormalities typically include subdural hematoma, although there have been reports of subdural hematoma that is not appreciated until autopsy.[38] This phenomenon has been described in the setting of severe cerebral swelling that affects the radiographic appearance of the subdural hemorrhage because of compression of the blood by the brain. In some cases, parenchymal contusion or brain lacerations may be found, but diffuse axonal injury is uncommon. Ischemic pathology found by immunohistochemistry is a prominent finding[6,25,39] External findings may be absent, but soft-tissue swelling, bruising, or a bulging fontanelle may be seen. New studies on cerebrospinal biomarkers indicate that chemicals released by the brain after injury may have future diagnostic or prognostic uses for this patient population, but their exact role remains incompletely understood at present.[40]

The physical examination should include the entire body, paying particular attention to the skin, abdominal, and skeletal systems to assess for additional signs of trauma. Consultation by a pediatric trauma surgeon is recommended to help with diagnosis and management of extracranial injuries.

Because of the variability in injury types and injury severity among patients, the spectrum of symptoms exhibited by the child can range from very subtle to severe alterations in consciousness or coma. The most commonly described symptoms are: vomiting, seizure, apnea, lethargy, and poor feeding. When symptoms are less specific, practitioners can miss the diagnosis, attributing the presentation to conditions, such as gastroenteritis, febrile seizures or flu-like illnesses.[41]

In addition to children who present with acute injuries, a particular challenge, diagnostically, is the child who presents with chronic subdural hematomas. These patients most often present with increasing head circumference. Some authors have pointed out that the most common cause of chronic subdural hematoma is trauma; however, chronic subdural hematoma has been associated with coagulopathies, structural abnormalities, and some rare genetic diseases.[42] For many children, no specific diagnosis is ever apparent. Work up for the etiology of a chronic subdural hematoma should include screening for appropriate medical conditions, as well as screening for child physical abuse, particularly as indicated by unrecognized skeletal injuries, the evaluation of which is detailed below. Referral to neurosurgery is standard, as surgical drainage or shunting is sometimes required.

Any finding suggestive of child physical abuse requires reporting to the appropriate social service or law enforcement agency. Most practitioners are aware of this and mandated reporting laws exist in all 50 states. The issue is worth readdressing; however, as research shows that some providers may not report physical abuse when suspected.[43]

DIFFERENTIAL DIAGNOSIS

There is a long list of medical conditions that have been cited in the literature as "mimics" of abusive head injury. The list of conditions associated with subdural/subarachnoid bleeding is extensive and includes the following: birth and other accidental trauma, congenital malformations, genetic and metabolic conditions, hematologic disorders, infectious diseases, toxins, complications of surgical intervention, vasculitides, oncologic processes, and nutritional deficiencies.[44]

A detailed discussion of all of these entities is beyond the scope of this text; however, some of the more commonly considered diagnoses will be reviewed. It should be noted, that most of those conditions can be differentiated from child abuse by careful consideration of the history, physical examination, and radiological or laboratory studies. Despite the existence of other conditions that can mimic child abuse, there should be strong consideration of a diagnosis of abuse in any case of a young child with a serious head injury who has no history of significant trauma.[28]

Asymptomatic intracranial hemorrhage after birth in normal, healthy newborns has been described. One study showed a prevalence of 26%.[45] Assisted deliveries may increase risk of injury, but intracranial hemorrhage has been documented with normal vaginal delivery. Birth-related subdural hematomas tend to present in an infratentorial location and typically disappear by 4 weeks of age.[46]

Congenital malformations, such as cerebral aneurysms and arteriovenous malformations, are relatively rare in young infants. Sagittal sinus thrombosis may occur in infants and lead to brain swelling, but this condition usually can be diagnosed by magnetic resonance (MR) imaging and MR venogram. Laboratory tests, radiographic findings, and patterns of nontraumatic causes of intracranial bleeding are usually distinguishable from that seen with abusive head trauma.

Some genetic and metabolic disorders can present with extra-axial hemorrhage, as well as with retinal hemorrhages or skeletal abnormalities. Practitioners should be aware of these conditions. Osteogenesis imperfecta and Menkes kinky hair disease can have skeletal abnormalities. Glutaric aciduria type I has some specific MR imaging but no associated skeletal findings. Universal screening for these and other diseases is not warranted and should be guided by the clinical presentation with input from the appropriate subspecialist. The incidence of most genetic diseases is lower than for child abuse and the possibility of comorbidity should be considered.[45]

Bleeding diatheses are a well-described group of inherited and acquired disorders that can cause intracranial hemorrhage. Coagulation studies should be done on all children with suspected abusive head injury. Screening labs should include prothrombin time, partial thromboplastin time, thrombin time, complete blood count with platelet count, fibrinogen and fibrin degradation products. Abnormal tests should prompt a hematology consult to guide further testing of platelet function or factor abnormalities. A history of prior episodes of bleeding, a positive family history, or a past history suggestive of vitamin K deficiency should direct more rapid communication with hematology specialists for specific treatment recommendations.

FORENSIC CONSIDERATIONS

After the diagnosis of abusive head trauma is confirmed, practitioners often face forensic questions from investigators with regard to identifying the mostly likely perpetrator, timing of injury, or alternative theories of injury. Generally, these types of questions are best left to the child abuse specialist if one is available. Radiology, pathology, and laboratory information, as well as determining the onset of symptoms, can help with questions of timing when a child was hurt.[47] However, it should be kept in mind that there are limits to the degree to which injuries can be timed or dated.

A number of studies support the generalization that children with abusive head injury are likely to be immediately symptomatic.[48] Most patients with acute subdural hematoma from large-force angular deceleration are immediately symptomatic, because the forces necessary to cause the rupture of parasagittal bridging veins also cause diffuse injury of the underlying brain.[49] The clinical scenario of an impact event followed by a "lucid interval" with later deterioration typically occurs in the setting of a clearly apparent contact event causing an expanding mass lesion, such as an epidural hematoma or subdural hemorrhage, with an associated contusion.[50,51] Second impact syndrome, a rare phenomenon usually occurring in athletes who sustain two concussive head injuries in series with potentially catastrophic brain swelling, has not been reported in young children.[52,53] In the setting of chronic subdural collections, it is well accepted that minor trauma can cause small volumes of acute rehemorrhaging into the subdural space; however, there is no evidence that significant rebleeding causing acute neurologic decline occurs spontaneously or with minor head injury.[54]

A history of a fall to account for brain injury to a child can also pose a diagnostic dilemma for practitioners attempting to differentiate between accidental and abusive head trauma. Chadwick, and colleagues[55] attempted to estimate the risk of death resulting from short falls of <1.5 m. Their review is the most comprehensive to date and reports a mortality rate of <0.48 deaths per 1 million young children per year. Other authors have cautioned that when severe injuries are seen with no history or with a history of a short fall, abuse should be seriously considered.[28] Arterial epidural hematomas can occur from low-height falls in infants and young children and can be life-threatening, but this type of injury is distinctly uncommon among abused children.[56]

In the case of fatal abusive head injury, the postmortem examination should be performed by a forensic pathologist who has experience in the standard procedures of dissection recommended in suspected child abuse cases.[57] Autopsy findings may reveal: contact injuries (skull fractures, soft tissue damage, or brain tissue contusions); inertial injuries (subdural hematomas, axonal injury, and tissue tears); injury at the craniocervical junction; secondary brain damage (hypoxic changes, cerebral edema); and associated injuries (bruises, skeletal injury, thoracoabdominal injury).[58] Axonal injury of the cervical spinal cord may be seen in children with abusive head trauma, suggesting a link to the pathophysiology of the condition. Some authors theorize that dysfunction of axons at the cervicomedullary junction causes apnea and hypoxia, which may contribute to global brain damage.[25,26,39]

ASSOCIATED INJURIES

In his 1974 paper, Caffey documented the association between head injury and long bone fractures.[14] It is worth emphasizing that child physical abuse is trauma. The possibility of multiple or occult injuries underscores the importance of a complete trauma assessment, including primary, secondary, and tertiary survey, by a well-coordinated, experienced trauma team.

As previously mentioned, the most common injuries seen in conjunction with abusive head trauma include soft tissue injury, skeletal injury, retinal hemorrhages and throcoabdominal injury, but genital injuries associated with sexual abuse, burns, and neglect may also be seen.[11,28,39] Rib fractures from squeezing of the chest and metaphyseal fractures from shearing type stresses on the end of the long bones may occur. There is generally no bruising over the fracture sites. More details regarding the radiologic evaluation of these injuries will be outlined in the following sections.

Retinal hemorrhages represent bleeding that occurs in or about the microscopic layers of the retina. The mechanism for retinal bleeding in the context of abusive head trauma has yet to be elucidated. Hemorrhaging may be preretinal, intraretinal and subretinal. Size and shape of the hemorrhagic lesions can also vary.[59,60] A detailed description or photograph of the findings during a dilated retinal examination by indirect ophthalmoscopy, preferably by an ophthalmologist, is essential in cases of suspected abusive head trauma. It is best if the eye exam is done early in the clinical course, before brain swelling or other factors might interfere with interpretation of the findings.[60,61]

The finding of retinal hemorrhages is not necessarily specific. They are observed in a variety of different medical conditions. Examples include vaginal birth (hemorrhages tend to be asymptomatic and disappear after about one month[62,63]), coagulopathy, accidental trauma, hypertension, increased intracranial pressure, papilledema, some metabolic diseases, toxins, infections, collagen disorders, and vasculitis.[61] It should be emphasized that the majority of the conditions in question can be ruled out based on history, physical examination, and lab testing.

The documented incidence of retinal hemorrhages in abusive head injury cases has ranged from 35%–100%, with most recent studies typically showing a rate of about 80%; a wide range of retinal hemorrhage characteristics, in terms of location and severity, have been described.[64–66] Severe, multilayered retinal hemorrhages in an otherwise healthy infant with a history of a low-height fall is considered by many in the field to be indicative of inflicted injury, and traumatic retinoschisis (where layers of the retina are cleaved forming a cystic cavity), optic nerve sheath hemorrhage, and vitreous or choroidal hemorrhage are ocular findings that should raise suspicion of significant trauma.[60,61,67,68] Several studies have demonstrated that retinal hemorrhages are a very rare occurrence after cardiopulmonary resuscitation and when seen, are typically minor when compared with child abuse cases.[69,70]

IMAGING

The appropriate use of radiography in the diagnosis of child abuse is well established. Because many injuries, including intracranial injuries, are unrecognized or present with subtle symptoms, imaging studies provide crucial information for diagnosis, treatment, and prognosis. Advancement in central nervous system radiographic techniques has improved our understanding of abusive head trauma. All infants and children with suspected inflicted head injury require brain imaging. Screening brain imaging of asymptomatic infants with a suspicion of maltreatment is recommended in children under the age of one year with facial injury, rib fractures, or multiple fractures and in any infant less than six months of age with any evidence of child physical abuse.[71]

Computed tomography (CT) is the mainstay for the diagnosis for intracranial injury in abusive head trauma, especially if a patient requires urgent evaluation. It is widely available in most facilities and it can be completed rapidly. CT is relatively sensitive for diagnosing intracranial hemorrhages and severe cerebral swelling or edema. Cerebral swelling on CT may manifest as loss of the gray–white matter differentiation, with relative sparing of the basal ganglia, cerebellum, thalami and brain stem. In this phenomenon, known as the "reversal sign," the above-mentioned structures appear brighter than the cortex.[72] The most common location for subdural hematoma in abusive head injury is in the parifalcine and tentorial regions or small collections over the cerebral convexities.[73,74] Despite its usefulness, CT may not detect shear injury, early cerebral edema, and skull fractures.[75] Cerebral edema may be patchy or involve one or both hemispheres, and may be seen as early as one hour post injury or may appear in a more delayed fashion over several days.[73,76–78]

Skeletal surveys are also important screening tools in any child under the age of 24 months with a suspicion of child physical abuse. In children age 2 to 5 years, skeletal survey should be reserved for cases where physical abuse is strongly suspected.[79] Any child with a confirmed abusive head injury should also have a skeletal survey. The skeletal survey consists of films of the extremities, skull and axial skeleton images, often times with multiple views. High-resolution techniques are recommended, either using special film or low-noise digital techniques. Inclusion of oblique views of the ribs may add to the detection of rib fractures. A "babygram," whereby the entirety of the infant's body is filmed in a single image, should be avoided, as it provides insufficient detail. Follow-up radiographs of the ribs to assess for healing fractures not seen in the acute phase or other areas suspicious for fracture may be helpful 2 to 3 weeks after the skeletal survey. Skeletal scintigraphy (bone scan) may used in place of radiographic skeletal survey. Scintigraphy can be more sensitive, but it is less specific and requires more radiation. It is more difficult and more expensive to perform. Follow-up radiography of any suspicious lesion is also required.[80]

Skull radiography is the modality of choice for the detection of skull fractures, although in some cases these may be better seen on CT scan, depending on the location of the fracture. Routine digital imaging may lower the rate of detection of bony injuries, and high resolution techniques may be needed.[81] All types of skull fracture can be seen with abusive injuries. Midline fractures, occipital fractures, multiple, complex, diastatic and depressed fractures are more suggestive of abuse if there is not a correlating history of an accident. Dating skull fractures can be difficult as compared with other bones, as the skull does not heal with typical callus formation.[82]

Magnetic resonance (MR) imaging is most frequently used to further delineate CT findings; however, some suggest that it may be an option for first-line evaluation of abusive head injury. MR imaging technology is changing rapidly, and newly developed sequences may give increasing information about the pathophysiology and evolution of injury.[75]

MR imaging and CT can be useful for determining age of hematomas. As a general rule on CT, acute blood appears hyperdense compared with cerebrospinal fluid (CSF) from time of injury to about 7–10 days; isodense collections indicate subacute blood between 7–10 days and 2–3 weeks; and chronic subdural collections are hypodense and occur from about 3 weeks onward.[83] The finding of mixed density lesions may indicate acute on chronic blood from either ongoing microhemorrhaging or reinjury (an important distinction). However, it is also recognized that because of tears in the arachnoid membrane and differential mixing and settling of blood components, heterogeneous, mixed density blood can be seen in the setting of acute injury, even in the very early hours after trauma.[84] For this reason, practitioners should avoid over-interpretation and reliance on imaging studies to date hematomas. Timing of injury can have important forensic implications, and efforts to estimate when a child was hurt should start with historical information regarding symptoms, severity of injury, and imaging studies with input from radiology colleagues. It should be understood that, even under the best circumstances, specifics about timing of injury may not be possible.

MANAGEMENT

An unrecognized insult to the brain, or one in which care is delayed, may result in decreased level of consciousness, hypoventilation, elevated intracranial pressure, seizure, or respiratory arrest.[85] Airway and ventilatory management are essential for optimizing conditions to limit progressive damage. However, much of the brain damage may occur early on in the disease process, caused by the cytotoxic effects of traumatic neuronal injury, hypoxia and cerebrovascular dysregulation.[85] In hospitalized children with injuries that are ultimately fatal, it is unclear whether any intervention significantly alters the outcome.[35] However, children with less severe injuries may benefit from aggressive intervention, which may limit damage. As mentioned, this intervention includes appropriate early recognition of more severe injuries; children who fail to show crying or grimacing typically have severe cortical injury.[36] Seizures are common and may be subclinical, so early intervention with anticonvulsants is generally recommended. Surgical intervention, including hemicraniectomy, has been advocated by some authors, particularly in the setting of predominantly unilateral injuries.[34,37]

OUTCOMES

Outcome studies regarding patients with abusive head injury have been historically difficult because of small sample sizes and methodologic issues, including a high loss to follow-up. Monitoring of outcome data has improved over the last decade and previously reported suspicions regarding prognosis have been confirmed. Overall, there is significant morbidity seen in survivors of abusive head injuries; outcomes range from mild learning disability to more severe physical or cognitive abnormalities and death.

Mortality ranges from 11% to 33% and almost two thirds of patients will have some neurologic sequelae.[86] Prognosis tends to correlate with the radiological severity of injury.[87] When comparing inflicted head injury with accidental head injury, patients in the abuse category have longer hospital stays, are more likely to have seizures, and more likely to have poor outcomes.[11,88] Neurologic manifestations of injury include heimplegia, quadriplegia, sight and hearing impairment, microcephaly, hydrocephalus and epilepsy.[86] Poor visual outcome is correlated with severe neurologic injury, and visual impairment is more often the result of brain injury than the presence of retinal hemorrhages.[66] Long-term behavioral, developmental and cognitive sequelae are also seen.[89]

PREVENTION

Prevention strategies include both general and specific approaches. Examples of general approaches include parenting support, which can be offered throughout childhood. At pediatric health supervision and immunization visits, health care providers can elicit concerns about behavior and offer age-appropriate anticipatory guidance. Parents can benefit from supportive community resources before abuse occurs.

Secondary prevention strategies focus on identifying high-risk families. When family dysfunction becomes apparent, early therapeutic intervention may be more effective than later intervention during adolescence. Early identification of mental health, family violence, and substance abuse issues is paramount. A broader view of child protection to include building on family strengths and youth mentoring may provide support that families need. In the event of fatal child abuse, state fatality review teams can assist communities in identifying specific needs.[90]

Unfortunately, few coordinated, evidence-based approaches to the prevention of abusive head trauma child abuse have been studied; however, one area of investigation has demonstrated positive effects. Neonatal education programs addressing new parent coping skills that focus on the stresses of infant crying have been shown to decrease the incidence of inflicted head injury.[7] More research is needed to see if this approach can be replicated. Preventive and therapeutic interventions need to be explored to find the most cost effective and humane strategies to approach the problem of child abuse. The results of such a strategy can only be evaluated by providing long-term follow-up for families. These approaches may be costly, but the cost of not protecting children may be higher.[10,11]

REFERENCES

1. Labbe J. Ambroise Iardieu: the man and his work on child maltreatment a century before Kempe. Child Abuse Negl 2005;29(4):311–24.
2. Kempe CH, Silverman FN, Steele BF, et al. The battered-child syndrome. JAMA 1962;181(1):105–12.
3. Guthkelch AK. Infantile subdural hematoma and its relationship to whiplash injuries. Br Med J 1971;2:430–1.
4. Caffey J. The whiplash shaken infant syndrome: manual shaking by the extremities with whiplash-induced intracranial and intraocular bleedings, linked with residual permanent brain damage and mental retardation. Pediatrics 1974;54: 396–403.
5. Bruce DA, Zimmerman RA. Shaken impact syndrome. Pediatr Ann 1989;18(8): 482–9.

6. Duhaime AC, Christian CW, Rorke LB, et al. Nonaccidental head injury in infants – the "Shaken Baby Syndrome." N Engl J Med 1998;338:1822–9.
7. Dias MS, Smith K, DeGuehery K, et al. Preventing abusive head trauma among infants and young children: a hospital-based, parent education program. Pediatrics 2005;115(4):e470–7.
8. Duhaime AC, Alario AJ, Lewander WJ, et al. Head injury in very young children: mechanisms, injury types and ophthalmologic findings in 100 hospitalized patients younger than 2 years of age. Pediatrics 1992;90:179–84.
9. Billmire EM, Myers PA. Serious head injury in infants: accident or abuse? Pediatrics 1985;75(2):340–2.
10. Libby AM, Sills MR, Thurston NK, et al. Costs of childhood physical abuse: comparing inflicted and unintentional and traumatic brain injuries. Pediatrics 2003;112:58–65.
11. Keenan HT, Runyan DK, Marshal SW, et al. A population-based study of inflicted traumatic brain injury in young children. JAMA 2003;290(5):621–6.
12. Barlow KM, Minns RA. Annual incidence of shaken impact syndrome in young children. Lancet 2000;356:1571–2.
13. Butchart A. Epidemiology the major missing element in the global response to child maltreatment. Am J Prev Med 2008;34(4S):S103–5.
14. Caffey J. Multiple fractures in the long bones of infants suffering from chronic subdural hematoma. AJR Am J Roentgenol 1946;56:163–73.
15. Silverman FN. Roentgen manifestations of unrecognized skeletal trauma in infants. Am J Roentgenol Radium Ther Nucl Med 1953;69:413–27.
16. Ommaya AK, Faas F, Yarnell P. Whiplash injury and brain damage: an experimental study. JAMA 1968;204:285–9.
17. Caffey J. On the theory and practice of shaking infants: its potential residual effects of permanent brain damage and mental retardation. Am J Dis Child 1972;124:161–9.
18. Ommaya AK, Corrao P, Letcher FS. Head injury in the chimpanzee. Part 1: biodynamics of traumatic unconsciousness. J Neurosurg 1973;39(2):152–66.
19. Duhaime AC, Gennarelli TG, Thibault LE, et al. The shaken baby syndrome. A clinical, pathological, and biomechanical study. J Neurosurg 1987;66:409–15.
20. Hahn YS, Chyung C, Barthel MJ, et al. Head injuries in children under 36 months of age. Childs Nerv Syst 1988;4:34–49.
21. Alexander R, Sato Y, Smith W, et al. Incidence of impact trauma with cranial injuries ascribed to shaking. Am J Dis Child 1990;144(6):724–6.
22. Prange MT, Coats B, Duhaime AC, et al. Anthropomorphic simulations of falls, shakes, and inflicted impacts in infants. J Neurosurg 2003;99(1):143–50.
23. Cory CZ, Jones B. Can shaking alone cause fatal brain injury? A biomechanical assessment of the Duhaime shaken baby syndrome model. Med Sci Law 2003; 43(4):317–33.
24. Hadley MN, Sonntag VKH, Rekate HL, et al. The infant whiplash-shake syndrome: a clinical and pathological study. Neurosurgery 1989;24:536–40.
25. Geddes JF, Hackshaw AK, Vowles GH, et al. Neuropathology of inflicted head injury in children. I. Patterns of brain damage. Brain 2001;124:1290–8.
26. Brennan LK, Rubin DM, Christian CW, et al. Neck injuries in young pediatric homicide victims. J Neurosurg, in press.
27. Hettler J, Greenes DS. Can the initial history predict whether a child with a head injury as been abused? Pediatrics 2003;111(3):602–7.
28. Reece RM, Sege R. Childhood head injuries: accidental or inflicted? Arch Pediatr Adolesc Med 2000;154(1):11–5.

29. Kairys SW, Alexander RC, Block RW, et al. American Academy of Pediatrics. Shaken baby syndrome: rotation cranial injuries—a technical report. Pediatrics 2001;108:206–10.

30. Case ME, Graham MA, Handy TC, et al. Position paper on fatal abusive head injuries in infants and young children. Am J Forensic Med Pathol 2001;22: 112–22.

31. Glick J, Staley K. Inflicted traumatic brain injury: advances in evaluation and collaborative diagnosis. Pediatr Neurosurg 2007;43:436–41.

32. Lee C, Barr RG, Catherine N, et al. Age-related incidence of publicly reported shaken baby syndrome cases: is crying a trigger for shaking? J Dev Behav Pediatr 2007;28:288–93.

33. Salehi-Had H, Brandt JK, Rosas AJ, et al. Findings in older children with abusive head injury: does shaken-child syndrome exist. Pediatrics 2006;117(5): e1039–44.

34. Feldman KW, Bethel R, Shugerman RP, et al. The cause of infant and toddler subdural hemorrhage: a prospective study. Pediatrics 2001;108:636–46.

35. Kesler H, Dias M, Shaffer M, et al. Demographics of abusive head trauma in the Commonwealth of Pennsylvania. J Neurosurg 2008;1:351–6.

36. Starling SP, Holden JR, Jenny C. Abusive head trauma: the relationship of perpetrators to their victims. Pediatrics 1995;95(2):259–62.

37. Starling SP, Patel S, Burke BL, et al. Analysis of perpetrator admissions to inflicted traumatic brain injury in children. Arch Pediatr Adolesc Med 2004;158(5):454–8.

38. Yair M, Isaac A, Louise C, et al. Shaken baby syndrome without intracranial hemorrhage on initial computed tomography. J AAPOS 2004;8(6):521–7.

39. Geddes JF, Hackshaw AK, Vowles GH, et al. Neuropathology of inflicted head injury in children. II. Microscopic brain injury in infants. Brain 2001;124: 1299–306.

40. Beers SR, Berger RP, Adelson PD. Neurocognitive outcome and serum biomarkers in inflicted versus non-inflicted traumatic brain injury in young children. J Neurotrauma 2007;24(1):97–105.

41. Jenny C, Hymel KP, Ritzen A, et al. Analysis of missed cases of abusive head trauma. JAMA 1999;281(7):621–6.

42. Swift DM, McBride L. Chronic subdural hematoma in children. Neurosurg Clin N Am 2000;11(3):439–46.

43. Jones J, Flaherty E, Binns H, et al. Clinicians' description of factors influencing their reporting of suspected child abuse: report of the child abuse reporting experience study. Pediatrics 2008;122(2):259–66.

44. Sirotnak A. Medical disorders that mimic abusive head trauma. In: Frasier L, Rauth-Farley K, Alexander R, et al, editors. Abusive head trauma in infants and children: a medical, legal and forensic reference. St. Louis (MO): G.W. Medical Publishing, Inc.; 2006. p. 191–226.

45. Looney CB, Smith JK, Merck LH, et al. Intracranial hemorrhage in asymptomatic neonates: prevalence on MR images and relationship to obstetric and neonatal risk factors. Radiology 2007;242(2):535–41.

46. Whitby EH, Griffiths PD, Rutter S, et al. Frequency and natural history of subdural haemmorrhages in babies and relation to obstetric factors. Lancet 2004;363: 846–51.

47. Boos SC. Abusive head trauma as a medical diagnosis. In: Frasier L, Rauth-Farley K, Alexander R, et al, editors. Abusive head trauma in infants and children: a medical, legal and forensic reference. St. Louis (MO): G.W. Medical Publishing, Inc.; 2006. p. 191–226.

48. Willman KY, Bank DE, Senac M, et al. Restricting the time of injury in fatal inflicted head injuries. Child Abuse Negl 1997;21(10):929–40.
49. Gennarelli TA, Thibault LE. Biomechanics of acute subdural hematoma. J Trauma 1982;22(8):680–6.
50. Duhaime AC. Epidural and subdural hematomas. In: Burg FD, Ingelfinger JR, Polin RA, et al, editors. Gellis and Kagan's current pediatric therapy. 16th edition. Philadelphia: W.B. Saunders; 1998. p. 436–8.
51. Starling SP. Head injury. In: Giardino AP, Alexander R, editors. Child maltreatment: a clinical guide and reference. 3rd edition. St. Louis (MO): G.W. Medical Publishing, Inc.; 2005. p. 37–62.
52. Saunders RL, Harbaugh RE. The second impact in catastrophic contact-sports head trauma. JAMA 1984;252(4):538–9.
53. Cantu RC. Criteria for return to competition after a closed head injury. In: Torg J, editor. Athletic injuries to the head, neck, and face. 2nd edition. St. Louis (MO): Mosby Year Book, Inc.; 1991. p. 323–30.
54. Kleinman PK, Barnes PD. Head trauma. In: Kleinman PK, editor. Diagnostic imaging of child abuse. 2nd edition. St. Louis (MO): Mosby; 1998. p. 285–342.
55. Chadwick DL, Bertocci G, Castillow E, et al. Annual risk of death resulting from short falls among young children: less than 1 in 1 million. Pediatrics 2008; 121(6):1213–24.
56. Shugerman RP, Paez A, Grossman DC, et al. Epidural hemorrhage: is it abuse? Pediatrics 1996;97(5):664–8.
57. Judkins AR, Hood IG, Mirchandani HG, et al. Technical communication. Rationale and technique for examination of nervous system in suspected infant victims of abuse. Am J Forensic Med Pathol 2004;25(1):29–32.
58. Gulino SP. Autopsy findings. In: Frasier L, Rauth-Farley K, Alexander R, et al, editors. Abusive head trauma in infants and children: a medical, legal and forensic reference. St. Louis (MO): G.W. Medical Publishing, Inc.; 2006. p. 297–313.
59. Gilliland MGF, Luckenbach MW, Chenier TC. Systemic and ocular findings in 169 prospectively studied child deaths: retinal hemorrhages usually mean child abuse. Forensic Sci Int 1994;68:117–32.
60. Kivlin JD. Manifestations of the shaken baby syndrome. Curr Opin Ophthalmol 2001;12:158–63.
61. Levin AV. Retinal haemorrhages and child abuse. In: David TJ, editor, Recent advances in paediatrics, 18. London: Churchill Livingstone; 2000. p. 151–219.
62. Emerson MV, Pieramici DJ, Stoessel KM, et al. Incidene and rate of disappearance of retinal hemorrhage in newborns. Ophthalmology 2001;108:36–9.
63. Hughes LA, May K, Talbot JF, et al. Incidence, distribution, and duration of birth related retinal hemorrhages: a prospective study. J AAPOS 2006;10:102–6.
64. Morad Y, Kim YM, Armstrong DC, et al. Correlations between retinal abnormalities and intracranial abnormalities in the shaken baby syndrome. Am J Ophthalmol 2002;134:354–9.
65. Pierre-Kahn V, Roche O, Dureau P, et al. Ophthalmologic findings in suspected child abuse victims with subdural hematomas. Ophthalmology 2003;110: 1718–23.
66. Kivlin JD, Simons KB, Lazoritz S, et al. Shaken baby syndrome. Ophthalmology 2000;107:1246–54.
67. Massicotte SJ, Folberg R, Torczynski E, et al. Vitreoretinal traction and perimacular retinal folds in the eyes of deliberately traumatized children. Ophthalmology 1991;98(7):1124–7.

68. Green MA, Lieberman G, Milroy CM. Ocular and cerebral trauma in non-acciental injury in infancy: underlying mechanisms and implication for paediatric practice. Br J Ophthalmol 1996;80:282–7.
69. Odom A, Shrist E, Kerr N, et al. Prevalence of retinal hemorrhages in pediatric patients after in hospital cardiopulmonary resuscitation: a prospective study. Pediatrics 1997;99:e3.
70. Kanter RK. Retinal hemorrhage after cardiopulmonary resuscitation or child abuse. J Pediatr 1986;108:430–2.
71. Rubin DM, Christian CW, Bilaniuk LT, et al. Occult head injury in high-risk abused children. Pediatrics 2003;111:1382–6.
72. Han BK, Towbin RB, de Courten-Myers G, et al. Reversal sign on CT: effect of anoxic/ischemic cerebral injury in children. Am J Roentgenol 1990;154:361–8.
73. Dias MS, Backstom J, Falk M, et al. Serial radiography in the infant shaken impact syndrome. Pediatr Neurosurg 1998;29(2):77–85.
74. Zimmerman RA, Bilaniuk LT, Bruce D, et al. Computed tomography of craniocerebral injury in the abused child. Radiology 1979;130(3):687–90.
75. Fernando S, Obaldo RE, Walsh IR, et al. Neuroimaging of nonaccidental head trauma: pitfalls and controversies. Pediatr Radiol 2007;38(8):827–38.
76. Steinbok P, Singhal A, Poskitt K, et al. Early hypodensity on computed tomographic scan of the brain in an accidental pediatric head injury. Neurosurgery 2007;60(4):689–95.
77. Gilles EE, Nelson MD Jr. Cerebral complications of nonaccidental head injury in childhood. Pediatr Neurol 1998;19(2):119–28.
78. Duhaime AC, Durham SR. Traumatic brain injury in infants: the phenomenon of subdural hemorrhage with hemispheric hypodensity ("Big Black Brain"). Prog Brain Res 2007;161:293–302.
79. American Academy of Pediatrics Section on Radiology. Diagnostic imaging of child abuse. Pediatrics 2000;105(6):1345–8.
80. Kleinman PK. Skeletal imaging strategies. In: Kleinman PK, editor. Diagnostic imaging of child abuse. 2nd edition. St. Louis (MO): Mosby; 1998. p. 237–41.
81. Kleinman PL, Kleinman PK, Savageau JA. Suspected infant abuse: radiographic skeletal survey practices in pediatric health care facilities. Radiology 2004; 233(2):477–85.
82. Demaerel P, Caseteels I, Wilms G. Cranial imaging in child abuse. Eur Radiol 2002;12:849–57.
83. Jaspan T. Current controversies in the interpretation of non-accidental head injury. Pediatr Radiol 2008;38(Suppl 3):S378–87.
84. Vinchon M, Noule N, Tchofo P, et al. Imaging of head injuries in infants: temporal correlates nd forensic implications for the diagnosis of child abuse. J Neurosurg 2004;101:44–52.
85. Gerber P, Coffman K. Nonaccidental head trauma in infants. Childs Nerv Syst 2007;23:499–507.
86. Jayawant S, Parr J. Outcome following subdural haemorrhages in infancy. Arch Dis Child 2007;92:343–7.
87. Bonnier C, Nassogne MC, Saint-Martin C, et al. Neuroimaging of intraparenchymal lesions predicts outcome in shaken baby syndrome. Pediatrics 2003;112(4): 808–14.
88. Hymel KP, Makaroff KL, Laskey A, et al. Mechanisms, clinical presentations, injuries, and outcomes from inflicted versus noninflicted head trauma during infancy: results of a prospective, multicentered, comparative study. Pediatrics 2007;119(5):923–9.

89. Barlow KM, Thomson E, Johnson D, et al. Late neurologic and cognitive sequelae of inflicted traumatic brain injury in infancy. Pediatrics 2005;116(2):e174–85.
90. Durfee MJ, Gellert GA, Tilton-Durfee D. Origins and clinical relevance of child death review teams. JAMA 1992;267(23):3172–5.

Retinal Hemorrhages: Advances in Understanding

Alex V. Levin, MD, MHSc

KEYWORDS

• Retinal hemorrhage • Child abuse • Shaken baby syndrome
• Abusive head trauma • Retinoschisis

Retinal hemorrhages are a cardinal manifestation of abusive head trauma character-ized by repetitive acceleration-deceleration forces with or without blunt head impact (shaken baby syndrome). Approximately 85% of affected children have retinal hemor-rhage, with just under two thirds having extensive, too numerous to count multilayered hemorrhages extending out to the edges of the retina (ora serrata) (**Fig. 1**).[1,2] Because there is a correlation between the severity of brain and eye injury,[1] the prevalence of retinal hemorrhage will be lower in children who survive neurologically intact and higher in those who die from their injuries.[3] Prevalence numbers are also affected by the inclusion of patients who sustain single acceleration-deceleration abusive impact head injury, because retinal hemorrhages are distinctly less common in this setting. Although nonophthalmologists are fairly good at indicating the presence or absence of retinal hemorrhage,[2,4] studies that rely on examinations by nonophthal-mologists must be analyzed cautiously.[5] Proper diagnosis of the ocular signs of abusive head injury requires pharmacologic dilation of the pupils and retinal examina-tion by an ophthalmologist familiar with this disorder.

Much has been learned about retinal hemorrhages since this syndrome was first described by Guthkelch[6] in 1971. Hundreds of articles from around the world have helped increased understanding of the importance of retinal hemorrhage as a diag-nostic indicator of abuse, particularly when the hemorrhages are extensive. This article is devoted to a discussion of the advances in knowledge regarding the documenta-tion, mechanisms, animal models, and outcomes of retinal hemorrhage.

DOCUMENTATION

Two major advancements have occurred in the ability to document the presence of retinal hemorrhage: (1) recognition of the need to detail the retinal findings and (2) retinal photography. The former speaks not only to documentation issues but also

Pediatric Ophthalmology and Ocular Genetics, Wills Eye Institute, 840 Walnut Street, 12th Floor, Philadelphia, PA 19107-5109, USA
E-mail address: alevin@willseye.org

Pediatr Clin N Am 56 (2009) 333–344
doi:10.1016/j.pcl.2009.02.003
0031-3955/09/$ – see front matter © 2009 Elsevier Inc. All rights reserved.

pediatric.theclinics.com

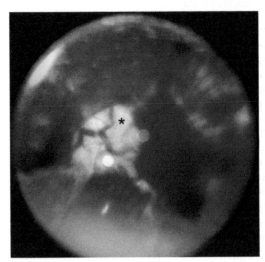

Fig. 1. Severe hemorrhagic retinopathy with too numerous to count retinal hemorrhages surrounding the optic nerve (*). Virtually no normal retina is visible due to the severity of the hemorrhages. In this patient the hemorrhages covered the entire retina extending out to the retinal periphery.

to differential diagnosis. A long list of systemic and ocular disorders (**Box 1**) is known to be associated with retinal hemorrhage. A nonspecific mild hemorrhagic retinopathy or a pattern specific for another diagnosis (eg, retinal infection) is usually present. In the case of the nonspecific retinal pattern, one may not be able to rule out or in abuse.

Box 1
Causes of infant retinal hemorrhage other than child abuse

Hypertension

Bleeding problems/leukemia

Meningitis/sepsis/endocarditis

Vasculitis

Cerebral aneurysm

Retinal diseases (eg, infection, hemangioma)

Carbon monoxide poisoning

Anemia

Hypoxia/hypotension

Papilledema/increased intracranial pressure

Glutaric aciduria

Osteogenesis imperfecta

Examinations in premature infants with retinopathy of prematurity

Extracorporeal membrane oxygenation

Hypo- or hypernatremia

Incomplete list. Diagnosis is usually easily made by history or systemic evaluation. Hemorrhages associated with these conditions are usually few in number and confined to the posterior pole; subretinal hemorrhage is extremely rare. Retinoschisis is not reported.

Fortunately, in almost every case, obvious historical, systemic, or ocular findings allow for a diagnosis and the elimination of a concern about abuse. Detailing the hemorrhagic retinopathy can offer specificity when considering etiology.

The retina is the inner lining of the eye, approximately the size of a postage stamp. The edges (ora serrata) are found just behind the iris for 360 degrees. The central visual axis through the pupil falls on the fovea, a small area of retina specialized for central visual acuity. The optic inserts nasal to the fovea, and its head (the optic disk) is visible on retinal examination. The area or retina surrounding the fovea is called the macula, which is, in turn, delimited by blood vessels that arise from the optic nerve and fan out on the retinal surface. The area encompassed by the major blood vessels (arcades) and containing the macula, fovea, optic nerve head, and some retina immediately around the nerve (peripapillary) is called the posterior pole (**Fig. 2**). The posterior pole can be visualized with a direct ophthalmoscope, but the retina beyond this region requires indirect ophthalmoscopy for proper visualization. The area of retina between the posterior pole and the region just leading to the ora (retinal periphery) is called the midperiphery. The vitreous gel that fills the eye is attached strongly in young children to the macula, the peripheral retina, and the retinal blood vessels coursing on the retinal surface before they dive deeper into retinal tissue.

Hemorrhages may occur on the surface of the retina (preretinal), under the retina (subretinal), or within the retinal tissue. In the latter circumstance, if the intraretinal hemorrhages are confined to the superficial nerve fiber layer of the retina, the hemorrhages take on a flame or splinter shape as the blood lays within the organized nerve fibers (**Fig. 3**). Hemorrhages deeper in the retinal tissue are more round or amorphous in shape and are called dot and blot hemorrhages arbitrarily based on the examiner's perception of their size. A particularly important form of hemorrhage is caused by the splitting of the retinal layers, with blood accumulating in the intervening space. This retinoschisis is sometimes accompanied by a circumlinear pleat or fold in the retina at its edges accompanied by hemorrhage or hypopigmentation (**Fig. 4**). Other than in abusive head injury, such lesions have only been reported in children under 5 years old in two cases of fatal crush injuries to the head[7,8] and in cases of severe fatal motor

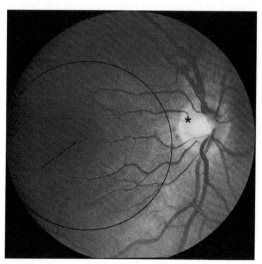

Fig. 2. Normal right eye posterior pole including fovea (*arrow*), macula (*within circle*), optic nerve (*), and retinal vessels emanating from the optic nerve.

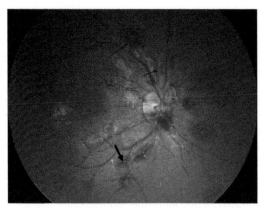

Fig. 3. Mild nonspecific retinal hemorrhage confined to the posterior pole. Short thin arrow indicates superficial intraretinal (flame) hemorrhage. Long thin arrow indicates preretinal hemorrhage. Thick arrow indicates blot intraretinal hemorrhage.

vehicle accidents.[9] These circumstances should be easily differentiated from abuse on historical grounds along with the presence of other characteristic injuries of these accidents. Hemorrhage may occur also in the vitreous in the absence of, or extending outward from, schisis cavities (see **Fig. 4**). Although there is no evidence that allows one to date the age of retinal hemorrhages in abusive head injury, the spreading of blood from a schisis cavity into the vitreous usually takes 1 to 3 days. As a result, patients with traumatic retinoschisis should be examined serially, because intervention for vitreous hemorrhage may be needed.

Retinal hemorrhages should be documented with a description of their numbers (ranging from none to too numerous to count), type, and extent. Diagnostic patterns should be recognized, such as the perivascular hemorrhage often seen in vasculitis or the classic radiating numerous intra- and preretinal hemorrhages of a central retinal vein occlusion. The presence or absence of retinoschisis is important to note as is the unilaterality or asymmetry of the hemorrhages between the two eyes, a finding that

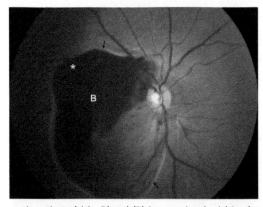

Fig. 4. Macular traumatic retinoschisis. Blood (B) is contained within the schisis cavity. Some blood is breaking through the internal limiting membrane wall of the cavity into the vitreous (*). Arrows indicate surrounding hypopigmented retinal fold at edge of schisis cavity.

can be seen in abusive head injury.[1] By avoiding use of the generic term *retinal hemorrhage* and instead detailing the findings, diagnostic specificity and sensitivity are enhanced.

Documentation can be achieved by good manual drawings with detailed descriptions. Photography is not required, but recent advancements have allowed photodocumentation which has the potential of being superior to hand drawings. Several cameras are available. The least expensive system is the Nidek camera (http://www.nidek-intl.com/fundus.html). Although the images are of lower quality, the cost of the camera, ease of use, and the ability to obtain images without pupillary dilation are favorable factors. The Kowa camera (http://www.kowa.co.jp/e-life/products/fc/index.htm) produces images[10] that have excellent quality. The camera has moderate expense but is technically difficult to use and does not yield a wide-angle view of the retina (see **Fig. 1**). RetCam photography (Clarity Medical Systems, Pleasanton, California, http://www.claritymsi.com)[10,11] is technically easier and wide angle but very expensive. RetCam images may also suffer from a "blackening" or loss of contrast when trying to capture hemorrhage and edge artifact (see **Fig. 3**). Patients can be photographed awake, but the eye must be still. More recently, techniques such as optical coherence tomography (OCT) have been used to document the vitreoretinal interface and schisis lesions.[12] This technique is not yet widely available for supine or noncompliant patients. MRI can sometimes detect retinal hemorrhage.[13] Most importantly, one must remember that photography, OCT, or MRI cannot replace a proper dilated clinical retinal examination by an ophthalmologist. In the setting of death before clinical examination, the fundus can be viewed for up to 72 hours in some cases, but postmortem documentation is a critical element and protocols have been established.[14–20]

MECHANISM

Understanding the mechanism of retinal hemorrhage, and in particular the severe hemorrhagic retinopathy that is seen almost exclusively in abusive head injury caused by repetitive acceleration-deceleration with or without blunt head impact (shaken baby syndrome), is tied to the ability to infer diagnostic implications. If one sees such hemorrhages and concludes that the child was likely abused, this conclusion must be based on a sound pathophysiologic link between the finding and a unique causality mechanism.

Using the commonality and even similarity (with the exception of retinoschisis and folds, which are absent) with the hemorrhages that can be seen in as many as 40% of normal children after birth,[3] consideration must be given to the effects of increased intracranial pressure or increased intrathoracic pressure. Because abused children may sustain rib fractures, it has been suggested that increased intrathoracic pressure could explain the presence of the retinal hemorrhages in those children. Hemorrhagic retinopathy is well known as a component of Purtscher syndrome, wherein adults who sustain severe chest crush injury have some retinal hemorrhage but, more importantly, a predominant and characteristic pattern of hexagonal white retinal patches which may be due to infarction, fat emboli from broken bones, or, in more recent studies, complement-mediated changes.[21,22] Purtscher retinopathy is only rarely seen in abusive head injury.[23] There appears to be no correlation between the presence of retinal hemorrhage and rib fracture.[1] Multiple studies examining the effects of chest compression as part of cardiopulmonary resuscitation have failed to demonstrate associated hemorrhagic retinopathy (or Purtscher syndrome) other than perhaps a few nonspecific retinal hemorrhages in the posterior pole.[24–28] Studies of other clinical scenarios involving increased intrathoracic pressure via Valsalva maneuvers in vomiting,[29] seizures,[30–32] or coughing[33] children also do not show significant retinal hemorrhaging.

Increased intracranial pressure with or without the presence of intracranial hemorrhage (Terson syndrome) can be associated with retinal hemorrhage in adults, particularly in those who experience acute elevations of pressure and subarachnoid hemorrhage. An increase in intracranial pressure in adults is associated with dilation of the optic nerve sheath,[34,35] whereas a study examining children with intracranial hemorrhage[36] and another investigating the relationship between increased intracranial pressure and retinal hemorrhage in abused children[1] failed to show significant relationships. If these factors do have a role in children, the influence is apparently small.

The postulated mechanism by which both increased intracranial and intrathoracic pressure would cause retinal hemorrhage is via the resistance or obstruction to venous outflow from the eye. Retinal venous obstruction is an easily recognized clinical presentation that is extremely uncommon in abusive head injury. The pattern of hemorrhages in the abused child is more random, not seemingly in keeping with venous distribution.

Further lack of support for a pathogenic mechanism invoking increased intracranial pressure in the pathogenesis of severe hemorrhagic retinopathy comes from two directions. First, papilledema is uncommon in abusive head injury (<10%),[1,2] despite the severity of the brain edema that may occur. Second, a multitude of studies of children with confirmed accidental head injury, many of whom experienced increased intracranial pressure (and intracranial hemorrhage), show a very low rate of retinal hemorrhage (<3% and in most studies 0%) which, when present, is characterized by a small number of pre- or intraretinal hemorrhages confined to the posterior pole or perhaps out to the midperiphery.[3,37–39] Although still confined largely to the posterior pole with a nonspecific appearance, retinal hemorrhage may be more common in patients with epidural hemorrhage.[40] In severe motor vehicle accidents, the rate of hemorrhage rises, and fatal cases have been reported with severe hemorrhagic retinopathy.[9,41] Similarly, fatal crush injury to the head has three times been reported to result in severe hemorrhages of the retina,[7,8,42] although such hemorrhages were not found in a larger study of similarly injured children.[43] The significance of those three cases remains obscure.[44] There appears to be something distinct about abusive head injury with repetitive acceleration-deceleration with or without head impact that results in a pattern of severe retinal hemorrhage.

Multiple lines of research have shown that the major factor in the causation of severe retinal hemorrhage is vitreoretinal traction.[3] Clinical evidence comes from the nature of the events described by confessed perpetrators,[45–47] the absence of such hemorrhagic retinopathy in single acceleration-deceleration (impact) trauma, and the pattern of hemorrhages, which correlates with the ocular anatomy of the young child wherein the vitreous is most adherent to blood vessels, the posterior pole in the area where the retinoschisis occurs, and the retinal periphery. Postmortem, the vitreous is often seen still attached to the apex of the perimacular retinal folds, consistent with the predicted causative traction.[48,49] In addition, researchers examining the orbital tissues behind the eye have demonstrated significantly higher amounts of hemorrhagic injury to those tissues, including the orbital fat, optic nerve dural sheath, and extraocular muscles.[50] It is believed that as the child is repeatedly accelerated and decelerated, the globe is translating in the orbit, causing damaging traction on the orbital structures. Intrascleral hemorrhage at another fulcrum point, the optic nerve-scleral junction, has also been observed.[50,51] Finite element analysis of the abusive repetitive acceleration-deceleration events also predicts tissue stress at the same area where retinal hemorrhage is observed in abused children.[52,53] The exact biochemical link between vitreoretinal traction and hemorrhage remains to be elucidated, although the importance of prostaglandins in the development of birth hemorrhage[54,55] and the presence of hemorrhage in the cranial nerve sheaths of abused children[50] suggest that traumatic autonomic denervation of the eye may have a role. This role is also supported by animal studies which indicate that shear at the vitreoretinal interface leads to disruption of vascular autoregulation with patulous and permeable retinal vessels.[56]

Although the importance of vitreoretinal traction makes intuitive sense and is well supported by research and clinical evidence, the role of other factors remains unknown but likely represents modulating influences that may determine variables such as the extent of hemorrhage in a given child. For example, although anemia, hypoxia, coagulopathy, and infection rarely cause retinal hemorrhages (and, when they do, produce nonspecific mild intraretinal hemorrhages),[3] perhaps these factors, which are commonly seen in abusive head injury, to some degree modulate the clinical retinal picture. These factors may also frequently accompany accidental head trauma, yet the rate of retinal hemorrhage remains low, suggesting once again the unique causative influence of repetitive acceleration-deceleration forces. Evidence from patients[57] with coagulopathy suggests that retinal hemorrhage is not likely even in the setting of trauma. Animal models of hypoxia do not demonstrate retinal hemorrhage.[58] One frequently quoted report suggests that hypoxia could cause retinal hemorrhage but did not involve any examination or research on ocular specimens.[59] This work was later retracted by one author under oath.[60] No studies have attempted to segregate these factors as dependent variables in either abusive or nonabusive head injury. Even when children present with multiple risk factors, severe hemorrhagic retinopathy should lead to serious consideration of abuse.[61]

Other factors also deserve further investigation. Thrombophilia, which is seen in approximately 5% of the North American population, is associated with retinal hemorrhage due to veno-occlusive disease in adults. Although the retinal vein obstruction pattern is absent in abusive head injury, the modulating effect of thrombophilia on the retinal response to accidental head injury is unknown. Likewise, the same can be said for vitamin C deficiency. Although not a significant cause of retinal hemorrhage even in severe deficiency, subclinical vitamin C deficiency has been reported in apparently healthy individuals,[62] and its effect in the setting of trauma is unknown. Unfortunately, prior studies have almost exclusively been performed measuring serum levels of vitamin C, a method that is unreliable and that should be replaced by measurement using lymphocytes.[63] Further research is needed with regards to both thrombophilia and vitamin C deficiency, but, until that time, laboratory studies remain neither useful nor interpretable. Although some have theorized a link between childhood immunization and retinal hemorrhage on the basis of a rise of histamine inducing vitamin C deficiency, there is little if any evidence to support such a theory.

ANIMAL MODELS

Modeling of the abusive injuries that lead to retinal hemorrhage has been fraught with physical and ethical challenges. Several groups, including our own, have investigated the ocular findings in rats or mice that have been mechanically shaken. Some investigators have reported retinal hemorrhages and, in those cases, the hemorrhages were apparently few in number (although not well described).[64–66] In our experiments (A. Levin, unpublished data, 2003), even with extreme and prolonged repetitive acceleration-deceleration forces at frequencies well beyond that which a human could create, we did not observe retinal hemorrhage except in one animal who also had blunt head trauma. We did observe distal optic nerve sheath hemorrhage. The greatest challenge to modeling the hemorrhagic retinopathy of abusive head injury becomes the magnitude of the forces needed when using such small animal eyes. In addition, the eyes are orientated more laterally and have less orbital development.

Larger animals have been shaken to death by other animals. In three examined animals, no retinal hemorrhages were found.[67] Once again, the challenge of the smaller eye may make the forces necessary to obtain injury too high. In addition, the shaking mechanism whereby the predator grasps the animal by the back of the neck may result in a dynamic that is not applicable to abusive head injury. Single lateral acceleration-deceleration of the pig head does not result in retinal hemorrhage, but further research with repetitive movement has not been completed.[68] Using this model, it has been shown that repeated acceleration-deceleration (two events separated by minutes) causes more severe brain injury than a single event.[69,70]

Remarkably, examination of woodpecker anatomy appears to have identified an ideal mechanism for protection against retinal injury.[71] The globe is encased in bone and affixed to surrounding fascial tissues, making it immobile in the orbit. Intrascleral cartilage and bone make the wall of the eye much stiffer than that of the notoriously soft human infant sclera. The vitreous is not attached to the retina. Nevertheless, the woodpecker has other adaptations which render it harder to extrapolate to human abusive injury. The skull is remarkably resistance to impact trauma, the strikes are anticipated, the strikes are mostly unidirectional, the eyes are very small, there are no retinal vessels, and the anatomic variations are seen in all birds. All birds do peck though. Perhaps the anatomic adaptations in the globe and orbit are one factor in allowing woodpeckers to evolve.

Studies using larger mammals, such as dogs, cats, or primates, with more developed orbital anatomy would be most fruitful. Our experience with a cat model in a city with the largest stray cat population and, secondarily, the largest endemic incidence of toxoplasmosis in the world where cats are routinely culled from the streets and slaughtered was unfortunately discontinued due to pressure from animal rights activists. The ethical challenges of performing research on larger mammals that better approximate the human infant need further examination and balance against the background of the scourge of abusive injury.

OUTCOMES

Retinal hemorrhage in of itself does not usually result in visual loss. Although the exact timing of hemorrhage resolution is unknown, the hemorrhages usually resolve without sequelae. Even macular retinoschisis has a surprisingly good prognosis, especially if only the internal limiting membrane of the retina is split away, as is usually the case. The central dome usually settles leaving no visible damage, although circumlinear hypopigmentary changes or retinal folds at the edge of the lesion may persist. These changes are visually insignificant. Retinal causes of visual loss in abusive head injury include full-thickness retinal detachment/avulsion, macular scarring/fibrosis, macular hole, and vitreous hemorrhage. In the last situation, surgery may be required to clear the visual axis. The role of surgical intervention in removing blood from schisis cavities is unknown. In both vitreous hemorrhage and macular schisis, the competing factors are the almost certain resolution with observation over time versus the amblyopia that is induced due to obstruction of the visual axis over that same time, particularly in the younger victim. Vitreous hemorrhage in particular may be a poor prognostic factor for ocular and systemic neurologic outcome.[72]

The most common causes of visual loss in abusive head injury are occipital cortical damage and optic nerve injury.[3] The former may occur as the result of direct brain contusion or counter coup injury affecting the occipital cortex or as a result of auto-infarction of the posterior circulation in the setting of severe cerebral edema. Optic nerve atrophy is also seen over time. Such change in the optic nerve is not caused by retinal hemorrhage or brain injury (except perhaps in the most severe and chronic cases in which retrograde optic nerve degeneration may be possible), suggesting the importance of direct optic nerve injury during the repetitive acceleration-deceleration injury.[50] Because there is no specific treatment for optic atrophy or cortical visual impairment, the vision prognosis for these children remains guarded.

SUMMARY

Retinal hemorrhage is a cardinal manifestation of abusive head injury characterized by repetitive acceleration-deceleration with or without blunt head impact. Describing the number, extent, type, and pattern of the hemorrhages aids in establishing a differential diagnosis. Mild posterior pole intra- and preretinal hemorrhage is nonspecific. Severe hemorrhagic retinopathy extending to the ora serrata, especially in the presence of macular retinoschisis with or without retinal folds, is highly associated with abusive head injury and appears to be a result of vitreoretinal traction and orbital injury. Documentation of the hemorrhages can be achieved manually or photographically. Animal models have yet to produce an exact model of this clinical entity. Although retinal hemorrhage rarely results in long-term vision compromise, the severity of the eye injury is correlated to the severity of brain injury, and poor visual outcomes may result from brain or optic nerve injury.

REFERENCES

1. Morad Y, Kim Y, Armstrong D, et al. Correlation between retinal abnormalities and intracranial abnormalities in the shaken baby syndrome. Am J Ophthalmol 2002; 134:354–9.
2. Kivlin J, Simons K, Lazoritz S, et al. Shaken baby syndrome. Ophthalmology 2000;107(7):1246–54.
3. Levin A. Retinal haemorrhage and child abuse. In: David T, editor, Recent advances in paediatrics, vol. 18. London: Churchill Livingstone; 2000. p. 151–219.
4. Morad Y, Kim Y, Mian M, et al. Non-ophthalmologists' accuracy in diagnosing retinal hemorrhages in the shaken baby syndrome. J Pediatr 2003;142(4):431–4.
5. Levin A. Fatal pediatric head injuries caused by short-distance falls. Am J Forensic Med Pathol 2001;22:417–8.
6. Guthkelch A. Infantile subdural haematoma and its relationship to whiplash injuries. Br Med J 1971;2:430–1.
7. Lantz PE, Sinal SH, Stanton CA, et al. Perimacular retinal folds from childhood head trauma. Br Med J 2004;328(7442):754–6.
8. Lueder GT, Turner JW, Paschall R. Perimacular retinal folds simulating nonacci-dental injury in an infant. Arch Ophthalmol 2006;124(12):1782–3.
9. Kivlin JD, Currie ML, Greenbaum VJ, et al. Retinal hemorrhages in children following fatal motor vehicle crashes: a case series. Arch Ophthalmol 2008; 126(6):800–4.
10. Levin AV. Child abuse. In: Levin A, Wilson T, editors. The Hospital for Sick Children's atlas of pediatric ophthalmology. Philadelphia: Lippincott Williams and Wilkins; 2007. p. 133–9.

11. Hoffman R, Mamalis N, Frasier L, et al. Ophthalmology: photographic examples. In: Frasier L, Rauth-Farley K, Alexander R, editors. Abusive head trauma in infants and children. St. Louis (MO): G.W. Medical Publishing; 2006. p. 151–9.

12. Scott AW, Farsiu S, Enyedi LB, et al. Imaging the infant retina with a hand-held spectral-domain optical coherence tomography device. Am J Ophthalmol 2008;147;364–73e2.

13. Altinok D, Saleem S, Zhang Z, et al. MR imaging findings of retinal hemorrhage in a case of nonaccidental trauma. Pediatr Radiol 2009;39(3):290–2.

14. Gilliland M, Levin A, Enzenauer R, et al. Guidelines for postmortem protocol for ocular investigation of sudden unexplained infant death and suspected physical child abuse. Am J Forensic Med Pathol 2007;28(4):323–9.

15. Parsons M, Start R. Necropsy techniques in ophthalmic pathology. J Clin Pathol 2001;54(6):417–27.

16. Matschke J, Puschel K, Glatzel M. Ocular pathology in shaken baby syndrome and other forms of infantile non-accidental head injury. Int J Legal Med 2008; [epub ahead of print].

17. Amberg R, Pollak S. Postmortem endoscopy of the ocular fundus: a valuable tool in forensic postmortem practice. Forensic Sci Int 2001;124:157–62.

18. Gilliland M, Folberg R. Retinal hemorrhages: replicating the clinician's view of the eye. Forensic Sci Int 1992;56(1):77–80.

19. Nolte K. Transillumination enhances photographs of retinal hemorrhages. J Forensic Sci 1997;42(5):935–6.

20. Lantz P, Adams G. Postmortem monocular indirect ophthalmoscopy. J Forensic Sci 2005;50(6):1450–2.

21. Agrawal A, McKibbin M. Purtscher's and Purtscher-like retinopathies: a review. Surv Ophthalmol 2006;51(2):129–36.

22. Agrawal A, McKibbin M. Purtscher's retinopathy: epidemiology, clinical features and outcome. Br J Ophthalmol 2007;91(11):1456–9.

23. Tomasi L, Rosman P. Purtscher retinopathy in the battered child syndrome. Am J Dis Child 1986;93:1335–7.

24. Gilliland M, Luckenbach M. Are retinal hemorrhages found after resuscitation attempts? A study of the eyes of 169 children. Am J Forensic Med Pathol 1993;14(3):187–92.

25. Goetting M, Sowa B. Retinal haemorrhage after cardiopulmonary resuscitation in children: an etiologic evaluation. Pediatrics 1990;85(4):585–8.

26. Fackler J, Berkowitz I, Green R. Retinal hemorrhage in newborn piglets following cardiopulmonary resuscitation. Am J Dis Child 1992;146:1294–6.

27. Kanter R. Retinal hemorrhage after cardiopulmonary resuscitation or child abuse. J Pediatr 1986;180:430–2.

28. Odom A, Christ E, Kerr N, et al. Prevalence of retinal hemorrhages in pediatric patients after in-hospital cardiopulmonary resuscitation: a prospective study. Pediatrics 1997;99(6):e3.

29. Herr S, Pierce M, Berger R, et al. Does Valsalva retinopathy occur in infants? An initial investigation in infants with vomiting caused by pyloric stenosis. Pediatrics 2004;113(6):1658–61.

30. Mei-Zahav M, Uziel Y, Raz J, et al. Convulsions and retinal haemorrhage: should we look further? Arch Dis Child 2002;86:334–5.

31. Sandramouli S, Robinson R, Tsalmoumas M, et al. Retinal hemorrhages and convulsions. Arch Dis Child 1997;76:449–51.

32. Tyagi A, Scotcher S, Kozeis N, et al. Can convulsions alone cause retinal haemorrhages in infants? Br J Ophthalmol 1998;82:659–60.

33. Goldman M, Dagan Z, Yair M, et al. Severe cough and retinal hemorrhage in infants and young children. J Pediatr 2006;148(6):835–6.
34. Gangemi M, Cennamo G, Maiuri F, et al. Echographic measurement of the optic nerve in patients with intracranial hypertension. Neurochirurgia (Stuttg) 1987;30:53–5.
35. Hansen H, Helmke K, Kunze K. Optic nerve sheath enlargement in acute intracranial hypertension. Neuroophthalmology 1994;14(6):345–54.
36. Schloff S, Mullaney P, Armstrong D, et al. Retinal findings in children with intracranial hemorrhage. Ophthalmology 2002;109(8):1472–6.
37. Bechtel K, Stoessel K, Leventhal JM, et al. Characteristics that distinguish accidental from abusive injury in hospitalized young children with head trauma. Pediatrics 2004;114(1):165–8.
38. Sturm V, Knecht PB, Landau K, et al. Rare retinal haemorrhages in translational accidental head trauma in children. Eye 2008; [epub ahead of print].
39. Pierre-Kahn V, Roche O, Dureau P, et al. Ophthalmologic findings in suspected child abuse victims with subdural hematomas. Ophthalmology 2003;110(9):1718–23.
40. Forbes B, Christina C, Cox M. Retinal hemorrhages in patients with epidural hematomas. J AAPOS 2008;12(2):177–80.
41. Vinchon M, Noizet O, Defoort-Dhellemmes S, et al. Infantile subdural hematoma due to traffic accidents. Pediatr Neurosurg 2002;37:245–53.
42. Obi E, Watts P. Are there any pathognomonic signs in shaken baby syndrome? J AAPOS 2007;11(1):99.
43. Gnanaraj L, Gilliland M, Yahya R, et al. Ocular manifestations of crush head injury in children. Eye, 2007;21:5–10.
44. Levin AV. Retinal hemorrhages of crush head injury: learning from outliers. Arch Ophthalmol 2006;124(12):1773–4.
45. Starling S, Patel S, Burke B, et al. Analysis of perpetrator admissions to inflicted traumatic brain injury in children. Arch Pediatr Adolesc Med 2004;158(5):454–8.
46. Leestma JE. Case analysis of brain-injured admittedly shaken infants: 54 cases, 1969–2001. Am J Forensic Med Pathol 2005;26(3):199–212.
47. Biron D, Shelton D. Perpetrator accounts in infant abusive head trauma brought about by a shaking event. Child Abuse Negl 2005;29(12):1347–58.
48. Massicotte S, Folberg R, Torczynski E, et al. Vitreoretinal traction and perimacular retinal folds in the eyes of deliberately traumatized children. Ophthalmology 1991;98(7):1124–7.
49. Emerson MV, Jakobs E, Green WR. Ocular autopsy and histopathologic features of child abuse. Ophthalmology 2007;114(7):1384–94.
50. Wygnanski-Jaffe T, Levin AV, Shafiq A, et al. Postmortem orbital findings in shaken baby syndrome. Am J Ophthalmol 2006;142(2):233–40.
51. Elner S, Elner V, Arnall M, et al. Ocular and associated systemic findings in suspected child abuse: a necropsy study. Arch Ophthalmol 1990;108:1094–101.
52. Rangarajan N, Kamalakkannan S, Hasija H, et al. Finite element model of ocular injury in shaken baby syndrome. J AAPOS, in press.
53. Bhola R, Cirovic S, Parson M, et al. Modeling of the eye and orbit to simulate Shaken Baby Syndrome [abstract]. Invest Ophthalmol Vis Sci 2005;46:e4090.
54. Gonzalez Viejo I, Ferrer Novella C, Pueyo Subias M, et al. Hemorrhagic retinopathy in newborns: frequency, form of presentation, associated factors and significance. Eur J Ophthalmol 1995;5(4):247–50.
55. Schoenfeld A, Buckman G, Nissenkorn I, et al. Retinal hemorrhages in the newborn following labor induced by oxytocin or dinoprostone. Arch Ophthalmol 1985;103:932–4.

56. Nagaoka T, Sakamoto T, Mori F, et al. The effect of nitric oxide on retinal blood flow during hypoxia in cats. Invest Ophthalmol Vis Sci 2002;43:3037–44.

57. Bray G, Luban N. Hemophilia presenting with intracranial hemorrhage: an approach to the infant with intracranial bleeding and coagulopathy. Am J Dis Child 1987;141:1215–7.

58. Ozbay D, Ozden S, Muftuoglu S, et al. Protective effect of ischemic preconditioning on retinal ischemia-reperfusion injury in rats. Can J Ophthalmol 2004;39:727–32.

59. Geddes J, Tasker R, Hackshaw A, et al. Dural haemorrhage in non-traumatic infant deaths: does it explain the bleeding in 'shaken baby syndrome'? Neuropathol Appl Neurobiol 2003;29:14–22.

60. Richards P, Bertocci G, Bonshek R, et al. Shaken baby syndrome. Arch Dis Child 2006;91:205–6.

61. Fenton S, Murray D, Thornton P, et al. Bilateral massive retinal hemorrhages in a 6-month-old infant: a diagnostic dilemma. Arch Ophthalmol 1999;117:1432–40.

62. Johnston CS, Solomon RE, Corte C. Vitamin C depletion is associated with alterations in blood histamine and plasma free carnitine in adults. J Am Coll Nutr 1996;15(6):586–91.

63. Emadi-Konjin P, Verjee Z, Levin A, et al. Measurement of intracellular vitamin C level in human lymphocytes by reverse phase high performance liquid chromatography (HPLC). Clin Biochem 2005;38:450–6.

64. Smith S, Andrus P, Gleason D, et al. Infant rat model of the shaken baby syndrome: preliminary characterization and evidence for the role of free radicals in cortical hemorrhaging and progressive neuronal degeneration. J Neurotrauma 1998;15:693–705.

65. Bonnier C, Mesples B, Gressens P. Animal models of shaken baby syndrome: revisiting the pathophysiology of this devastating injury. Pediatr Rehabil 2004;7(3):165–71.

66. Bonnier C, Mesples B, Carpentier S, et al. Delayed white matter injury in a murine model of shaken baby syndrome. Brain Pathol 2002;12:320–8.

67. Serbanescu I, Brown S, Ramsay D, et al. Natural animal shaking: a model for inflicted neurotrauma in children? Eye 2008;22(7):715–7.

68. Binenbaum G, Forbes B, Reghupathi R, et al. Animal model to study retinal hemorrhages in a non-impact brain injury. J AAPOS 2007;11(1):84–5.

69. Huh JW, Widing AG, Raghupathi R. Repetitive mild non-contusive brain trauma in immature rats exacerbates traumatic axonal injury and axonal calpain activation: a preliminary report. J Neurotrauma 2007;24(1):15–27.

70. Raghupathi R, Mehr MF, Helfaer MA, et al. Traumatic axonal injury is exacerbated following repetitive closed head injury in the neonatal pig. J Neurotrauma 2004;21(3):307–16.

71. Wygnanski-Jaffe T, Murphy C, Smith C, et al. Protective ocular mechanisms in woodpeckers. Eye 2007;21:83–9.

72. Matthews G, Das A. Dense vitreous hemorrhages predict poor visual and neurological prognosis in infants with shaken baby syndrome. J Pediatr Ophthalmol Strabismus 1996;33:260–5.

Substance Abuse and Child Maltreatment

Kathryn Wells, MD, FAAP[a,b,c,]*

KEYWORDS

• Substance abuse • Child maltreatment

Pediatricians and other medical providers caring for children need to be aware of the dynamics in the significant relationship between substance abuse and child maltreatment. A caregiver's use and abuse of alcohol, marijuana, heroin, cocaine, methamphetamine, and other drugs place the child at risk in multiple ways. Members of the medical community need to understand these risks because the medical community plays a unique and important role in identifying and caring for these children. Data from the Substance Abuse and Mental Health Services Administration's 2007 National Survey on Drug Abuse and Health indicate that an estimated 19.9 million Americans aged 12 or older (8% of the population) were current users of illicit drugs, including marijuana/hashish, cocaine, heroin, hallucinogens, inhalants, and prescription-type psychotherapeutics used nonmedically.[1] Additionally, 126.8 million people, 51.1% of the population aged 12 or older, reported being current drinkers of alcohol and 23.3% (57.8 million) reported that they regularly participated in binge drinking, while 6.9% (17 million) of the population reported heavy drinking. Substance abuse includes the abuse of legal drugs (eg, alcohol, prescription drugs, over-the-counter drugs) as well as the use of illegal drugs (eg, cocaine, heroin, marijuana, and methamphetamines). The abuse of legal substances may be as detrimental to parental functioning as abuse of illicit substances. Additionally, many substance abusers are also polysubstance users and the compounded effect of the abuse of multiple substances may be difficult to measure. Finally, there are often other interrelated social features, such as untreated mental illness, trauma history, and domestic violence, affecting these families.

EPIDEMIOLOGY

Research has confirmed a strong connection between substance abuse and child maltreatment.[2,3] In one study that controlled for many variables, children whose

[a] Community Health Services, Denver Health, Denver, CO, USA
[b] Department of Pediatrics, University of Colorado School of Medicine, Aurora, CO, USA
[c] Denver Family Crisis Center, 2929 West 10th Avenue, Denver, CO 80204, USA
* Denver Family Crisis Center, 2929 West 10th Avenue, Denver, CO 80204.
E-mail address: Kathryn.wells@dhha.org

Pediatr Clin N Am 56 (2009) 345–362
doi:10.1016/j.pcl.2009.01.006
0031-3955/09/$ – see front matter © 2009 Elsevier Inc. All rights reserved.

parents were abusing substances were found to be 2.7 times more likely to be abused and 4.2 times more likely to be neglected than other children whose parents were not substance abusers.[3-5] In a 1998 survey of the 50 state child protection service agencies, the National Committee to Prevent Child Abuse (now Prevent Child Abuse America) reported that 85% of the states indicated that substance abuse was one of the two leading problems exhibited by families reported for child maltreatment[6] with poverty being the other most frequently reported issue. Review of juvenile court data in one study showed that, in 43% of cases of serious child abuse or neglect, at least one parent had a documented problem with either alcohol or drugs and instances of substance abuse allegedly took place in 50% of the cases.[7] This study also showed that parents with documented substance abuse, in comparison with parents with no documented substance abuse, were more likely to have been previously charged with child maltreatment and were also more likely to be rated as high risk to their children, more likely to reject court-ordered services, and were more likely to have their children permanently removed. Parental substance abuse has been linked to the most serious outcomes of all cases of child maltreatment, including fatalities. Data by Reid and colleagues[8] indicate that substance abuse by caregivers is associated with as many as two thirds of all cases of child maltreatment fatalities.[8] In this study, 51% of these deaths involved physical abuse while 44% involved neglect and 5% involved multiple forms of child maltreatment.

SUBSTANCE ABUSE AS RISK FOR CHILD MALTREATMENT

The combined stresses of substance abuse and the demands for the routine care of infants and children can create a volatile or otherwise vulnerable environment in which neglect or physical abuse can occur. Parents or caregivers who are acutely intoxicated or withdrawing from drugs or alcohol will not respond appropriately to the cues an infant or child gives for both physical and social interactive nurturing. A parent or caregiver who abuses substances has impaired judgment and priorities and is unable to provide the consistent care, supervision, and guidance that children need. Additionally, these homes are often plagued with other problems, including physical or mental illness; poor parenting skills; domestic violence; involvement of caregivers with drugs, alcohol, and criminal activity; and lack of such resources as money, time, energy, and emotional support for the children. Finally, many drugs of abuse make adult caregivers violent, paranoid, and angry, creating a situation where the caregiver is more prone to injure or neglect their children.[9] For all these reasons, substance abuse is clearly a critical factor in child welfare.[10] Along with previous referrals to child protective services, history of domestic violence, history of caregiver child abuse and neglect as a child, and caregiver impairments, the presence of substance abuse in the home strongly correlates with the recurrence of child maltreatment.[11]

To break the cycles of addiction and child maltreatment, children at risk in environments where substance abuse takes place must be identified. Children who grow up in homes where substance abuse is an issue have poorer outcomes (behaviorally, psychologically, socially, and physically) than children whose parents or caregivers do not abuse substances. Without intervention, these children are at increased risk of substance abuse themselves. Children who were abused during their childhood have a greater risk of substance abuse later in life, highlighting the importance of breaking this cycle of addiction.[12]

Children in homes where alcohol is being abused or drugs are being used are exposed to many risks ranging from prenatal exposure and the effects it may have on the fetus to potential exposure to the drugs themselves and exposure to a violent and chaotic environment. Affected families must be identified so that the children can be properly evaluated and an ongoing safety plan can be established.

PRENATAL DRUG EXPOSURE: EFFECTS ON MOTHER AND FETUS

Prenatal drug exposure may be accompanied by additional effects on the infant's health before birth and in the immediate neonatal period. Many of these children are not identified because their mothers do not disclose their substance abuse for fear of prosecution or fear of losing custody of their children. However, during pregnancy and soon after birth may be the most effective time for intervention, as motherhood is often the only legitimate social role that is valued by drug-dependent women, and most women in treatment are quite concerned about how their substance abuse affects their children. Therefore, pregnancy and motherhood are times of increased motivation for treatment. Studies that have tried to assess the direct risks to children exposed to drugs in utero have found it difficult to dissociate the negative effects of the actual drug exposure from the negative effects of other variables, including poor prenatal care, poor prenatal nutrition, prematurity, and an adverse postnatal environment. However, the identification of maternal substance abuse in the prenatal period should serve as a red flag for potential risks in the postnatal environment. Recent studies have shown that drug-exposed infants may be at greater risk of harm in the postnatal environment than in the prenatal environment. After birth, children have been shown to be at increased risks for child maltreatment after birth. One study showed that infants exposed to drugs in utero were more likely than other infants to be reported as abused or neglected (30.2%) and this later results in substantiated cases of abuse and neglect (19.9%), a rate that was two to three times that of other children in the same geographic area.[13] Therefore, it is important for prenatal exposure to drugs or alcohol to be identified not only for medical treatment purposes but also as an opportunity to address the many other issues the family may be confronting.

Pregnant women who are substance abusers are at far greater risk than other pregnant women for a range of medical problems. They are at greater risk for many infections, including HIV, sexually transmitted diseases, tuberculosis, hepatitis B and C, endocarditis, syphilis, pneumonia, and tuberculosis. In addition, they may display nutritional deficiencies and anemia, as well as toxin-induced organ damage to the heart (eg, contraction band necrosis, cardiomegaly, cardiomyopathy), lungs, liver, gastrointestinal tract, or kidneys. Additional obstetrical complications include bacteremia, septicemia, cellulitis, edema, abscesses, hypertension, tetanus, urinary tract infections, amnionitis, chorioamnionitis, placental insufficiency, eclampsia, gestational diabetes, premature labor and rupture of the membranes, abruptio placentae, spontaneous abortion, intrauterine growth retardation, intrauterine death, premature birth, and postpartum hemorrhage.[14] Many women who are using substances do not seek out adequate prenatal care, which places the infant and the mother at increased risk for complications. Mothers who do not receive prenatal care are more likely to give birth to low–birth-weight infants, which places them at increased risk of death and other complications during the first several weeks of life. Additionally, these babies may be born outside the hospital in an uncontrolled setting, placing them at further risk.

The potential effects of maternal substance abuse on the fetus and infant depend greatly on the substance being used, the frequency of use, the duration of use, and the quantity used. Often, women use multiple chemicals, which may interact with one another, placing the infant at even greater risk. Neonatal complications of maternal substance abuse include decreased birth weight, body length, and head circumference; possible impairment of brain development; intrauterine growth retardation; fetal distress; immune deficiency; hyperbilirubinemia; hypoglycemia; intracranial hemorrhage; neonatal abstinence syndrome; pneumonia; infections; intrauterine death; and increased risk for death from sudden infant death syndrome.[15] Because these infants are at risk of prematurity, they frequently have low–birth weights and are at increased risk for a host of related problems. These complications may include breathing problems requiring mechanical ventilation and oxygen, intracranial hemorrhage, overwhelming infections requiring antibiotics, and poor feeding, often requiring artificial feeding assistance. Prenatal substance abuse can lead to specific medical and developmental problems for the child. For example, depending on the gestational age of the fetus when the drug was used, there may be congenital abnormalities, such as those involving the neurologic, pulmonary, renal, or digestive systems. Additionally, a great deal of research has shown long-term developmental and behavioral issues in children exposed to drugs and alcohol in utero. Recently, volumetric MRIs assessing the effects of intrauterine exposures to cocaine, alcohol, and cigarettes on infants' brains have shown that these exposures are individually related to reduced head circumference, cortical gray matter, and total parenchymal volumes at school age.[16]

Studies over the last several years have clearly shown that alcohol ingested by the pregnant woman crosses the placenta to the fetus. Therefore, any amount of alcohol ingested during pregnancy may harm the infant. The latest research shows that no amount of alcohol is safe to ingest while pregnant. Infants exposed in utero to alcohol are at risk for fetal alcohol spectrum disorder, which occurs in 1 out of 200 births worldwide and accounts for 5% of all congenital anomalies, as well as 10% to 20% of all cases of mental retardation. Fetal alcohol spectrum disorder constitutes a wide range of disorders, the most serious of which is fetal alcohol syndrome (FAS), which is known to be the leading preventable cause of mental retardation and birth defects. FAS is a constellation of physical characteristics and behavioral and developmental problems that children who were exposed to alcohol in utero may display. The unique infant traits associated with this syndrome include such physical characteristics as an abnormally small head, a low nasal bridge, small eyes, a flat midface, a short nose, and a thin upper lip. The syndrome is also associated with irritability in infancy, low–birth weight or sustained smallness in size for age, moderate intellectual impairment, and frequent hyperactivity and attentional impairments in childhood. Many of these children also have developmental delays, hypotonia, and motor problems and may develop a seizure disorder.

Children with fetal alcohol effects are those who were exposed to alcohol in utero and display the same the behavioral and developmental difficulties as children with FAS, but who don't display the physical/facial characteristics of children with FAS. Clearly prenatal exposure to alcohol has a broad and profound impact on the long-term development of children with fetal alcohol effects. One recent study that controlled for various prenatal and postnatal factors showed that maternal consumption of less than one drink per week during the first trimester of pregnancy was independently associated with clinically significant mental health outcomes in girls at 47 months as measured by the Strengths and Difficulties Questionnaire, which is a well-validated measure of childhood mental health.[17]

Marijuana exposure in utero has been linked to infants displaying increased tremors, an exaggerated startle reflex, poorer habituation to visual stimuli,[18] a high-pitched cry,[19] and reduced quiet sleep.[20] A recent study of adolescent mothers who used marijuana during pregnancy showed that prenatal exposure was associated with subtle behavioral changes in the infants, especially in terms of arousal, regulation, and excitability.[21] This may potentially interfere with the infant's ability to bond with his or her mother. Additionally, effects on later stages of development have been shown. These effects include decreased memory and verbal functions at 3 and 4 years of age; poor attention and impulsivity in children aged 6 years; and reduced head circumference, visual analysis, and hypothesis testing at 9 to 12 years of age.[22]

Addiction to opioids, such as heroin and methadone, is also associated with all the prematurity and low–birth-weight problems described for prenatal exposure to alcohol and other drugs. In addition, studies show that 55% to 94% of infants exposed prenatally to opiates experience some degree of life-threatening withdrawal symptoms shortly after birth.[23] These symptoms, collectively called the neonatal abstinence syndrome, include an increased Moro/startle reflex, tremors, irritability, inability to self-quiet, poor feeding, abnormal sleep patterns, diarrhea, fever, and seizures. The infant may also display central nervous system hyperactivity, high-pitched cry, increased muscle tone, gastrointestinal dysfunction, respiratory distress, and autonomic symptoms, including yawning, sneezing, mottling, and fever. Because of the short half-life of the drug, most infants exposed to opioids prenatally display these symptoms only during the first 24 hours of life.[24] If the mother has been on methadone maintenance during the pregnancy and has been receiving regular prenatal care, the risk of obstetric and fetal complications is reduced. However, for infants of mothers on methadone, neonatal abstinence syndrome may be more severe and may be delayed 24 to 48 hours because of the drug's extended half-life.[24] Additionally, symptoms in the infant may last from a few days up to 8 weeks.[25] Limited longitudinal data suggest that children born to heroin-using or methadone-maintained women appear to have normal mental and motor development at the time they enter school.[15]

Numerous studies have looked at the effect of prenatal exposure to such stimulants as cocaine and methamphetamine. In utero exposure to cocaine has been linked to intrauterine growth retardation, microcephaly, prematurity, hypertension, central nervous system hemorrhage, stroke, genitourinary abnormalities, increased risk for sudden infant death syndrome and HIV, and necrotizing enterocolitis.[26] These infants may also display increased irritability, tremulousness, and state lability, which is felt to be due to increased catecholamine activity and may interfere with maternal and infant bonding.[24] An abstinence syndrome that may occur 2 to 3 days after birth has been described but is less clear than that defined in opiate exposure. No well-defined scoring system to measure the syndrome has been established. Some studies have indicated that prenatal cocaine exposure is linked with decreased head circumference, lower IQ scores, and increased behavioral problems by 3 years of age.[27] Studies have also shown a link between prenatal cocaine exposure and slower development of language skills during the first 6 years of life.[28] One recent study found that prenatal cocaine exposure has a negative impact on the trajectories of childhood behavior outcomes with added negative effects if that prenatal exposure occurs along with prenatal and postnatal exposure to tobacco and alcohol.[29] Although there are some potential adverse effects on the fetus from prenatal exposure to cocaine, the assumptions in the 1980s and 1990s that all exposed children would have universally bad outcomes have been disproved and the impact of postnatal environment has been given a greater role in the ultimate outcomes for these children. Therefore, early identification of exposure and initiation of services as indicated are important to improve the prospects for these children.

Studies on the effects of prenatal exposure to methamphetamine are in their early phases. The first large-scale multisite investigation to report the prevalence of methamphetamine use during pregnancy in high-use areas of the United States has recently begun and initial findings have indicated that 5.2% of the women used methamphetamine at some point in their pregnancy.[30] Early results from this study confirm that prenatal methamphetamine use is associated with fetal growth restriction and a 3.5-fold increased risk of an infant being small for gestational age.[31] This large study will continue to investigate outcomes associated with prenatal methamphetamine exposure. However, it is now believed that the effects may be similar to the problems found in cocaine-exposed babies and may include placental abruption; arrhythmias; prematurity; in utero growth retardation; brain abnormalities, including hemorrhage and infarction; a variety of birth defects (particularly gastrointestinal); and poor sucking and feeding difficulties after birth. While cocaine-exposed infants are noted to be quite irritable initially, methamphetamine-exposed infants tend to be sleepy and lethargic for the first few weeks, often to the point of not waking to feed. After the first few weeks, they may resemble cocaine-exposed infants, becoming quite jittery, having a shrill cry, and often startling at the slightest stimulation. This behavior pattern is now believed to be due to initial catecholamine depletion followed by increased catecholamine activity. The risk of sudden infant death syndrome is reported to be higher in cocaine- and methamphetamine-exposed[32] babies, although there are other confounding variables, such as inadequate prenatal care and concomitant cigarette smoking.

Additionally, these children are felt to display long-term delays in development. One study showed a significant correlation between the extent of amphetamine exposure and impaired psychometric testing, including behavioral and adjustment problems,[33] while another study showed later developmental effects, including poor state control, difficulty with habituation, and impairment in reflexes.[34] One area that is concerning but not yet researched is the effect of prenatal exposure to methamphetamine manufacturing on the fetus. Some of the components of the manufacturing process are organic solvents and one study found that prenatal exposure to such substances is associated with selective visual deficits.[35]

ENVIRONMENTAL DANGERS
Family Functioning

Research continues in the area of family functioning in environments of drug and alcohol addiction. However, it is already clear that the effects of prenatal drug or alcohol exposure are difficult to separate from the poor functioning and environmental conditions in which many of these families exist. Therefore, potentially more important than the individual medical and developmental complications of the prenatal drug or alcohol exposure is the correlation of prenatal substance abuse with poor outcomes in relation to postnatal outcomes. Alcohol- and drug-related cases are more likely to result in foster care than are other child welfare cases. Once in foster care, children whose parents or caregivers have substance abuse problems tend to remain in care for longer periods of time. This raises particular challenges given the many conflicting timelines imposed on families dealing with these issues. The child has a developmental timeline in which growth and development occurs dramatically over the first 3 years of his or her life, making this a critical time for consistency. The timeline for substance addiction recovery for the parent is a lifetime, with much intervention and support needed in the early stages of the recovery. Additionally, there are guidelines imposed on families involved in the child welfare system, requiring a permanency plan to be established by 1 year after placement of the child. Finally, other temporary financial-assistance timelines play a role in meeting families' needs.[10]

Child Abuse and Neglect

Because of a multitude of factors, infants born to mothers with substance-abuse issues are at a greater risk for child abuse and neglect. Many infants born to substance-abusing mothers are left with alternative caregivers for extended periods of time and are often abandoned. In some cases, their mothers die early from problems related to substance use or violence. Those infants who go home with a parent are at an increased risk from medical and environmental neglect because of special medical needs. These children, often fussy and difficult to console, may easily frustrate any caregiver. If this situation is coupled with the caregiver's use of a substance to deal with the stress, the risk to the child is further increased. For example, a small infant in communicating its needs by crying can cause additional frustrations for a caregiver who uses drugs or alcohol to cope, leading that caregiver to use more drugs to temper his or her anxiety. Unfortunately, the use of drugs may lead to further difficulty with anger and the caregiver may finally become so frustrated and upset that he or she may harm the infant. The use of drugs and alcohol can be associated with a lower frustration threshold. One study showed that there was an increase of maltreatment in children born to mothers who used cocaine during pregnancy, but when socioeconomic factors were controlled for, it was found that those factors partially accounted for the increased risk of maltreatment. It was concluded that the mother's use of cocaine was more likely a marker of increased risk than a single explanatory variable.[36]

Exposures and Ingestions

Danger to children of exposure to drugs extends beyond the prenatal period. Homes where illegal drugs are being used or alcohol is being abused present many environmental risks for children. Children may come into direct contact with the drugs. For example, they may breathe air containing marijuana, cocaine, or methamphetamine smoke, or they may find the drugs themselves and ingest them. Additionally, these environments may be chaotic and expose the child to physical hazards, such as unsafe and unsanitary conditions, domestic violence, pornography, and criminal activity, including use of firearms and other weapons. More importantly, these children are at risk of direct physical abuse and overt neglect.

Direct exposure of children to substances of abuse after birth is an important potential risk that is often overlooked. An infant breastfed by a mother who continues to use drugs or alcohol will continue to be exposed to the drug, which may have devastating consequences. Several studies have shown dangerously high levels of alcohol and illegal drugs in infants breastfed by mothers who were active substance abusers.[37–39] Additionally, to date, at least two women have been convicted of giving their infants methamphetamine through the breast milk, which was believed to ultimately result in the infants' deaths.[40] Each mother should be told clearly that breastfeeding while continuing to use drugs and alcohol is not safe for infants.

Children living in homes where drugs are being abused may accidentally ingest substances left accessible to them or may become victim to passive exposure to marijuana, methamphetamine, phencyclidine (PCP), and crack cocaine when smoked by caregivers in their presence.[41–43] Exposure to alcohol, cocaine, methamphetamine, and PCP may produce signs and symptoms of intoxication. These signs and symptoms may include lethargy, vomiting, seizures, apnea, coma, and death.[44] Although children may ingest alcohol left accessible in the home, several studies have provided disturbing evidence of occult illicit drug exposure in children. One study looked at 460 children between 1 and 60 months who presented to an urban pediatric emergency department for routine complaints and found that benzoylecgognine (a metabolite of cocaine) was found in 5.4% of the patient's urine samples using usual screening techniques.[45] Another children's hospital study found that 5% of children screened had urine specimens containing cocaine or its metabolite,[46] while yet another study found a 2.4% (6 of 250) positive rate of drugs screens for benzoylecgognine, 4 in children under 1 year and all in children younger than 24 months. Possible routes of exposure considered were breastfeeding, intentional administration, accidental ingestion, and passive inhalation. Another study used a more sensitive radioimmunoassay technique to analyze 124 urine samples of children presenting for routine concerns to an emergency department. That study found that 36.3% were positive for cocaine or its metabolite.[47] Additionally, it was found that these children had a higher rate of upper- and lower-respiratory symptoms, which may be related to passive exposure and may suggest that these children have increased medical needs.[47]

Most cases of accidental ingestions in the literature are related to cocaine and methamphetamine ingestions. One article reported four cases of children aged 4 months to 3 years who presented with seizures due to cocaine ingestion,[48] while another described a 9-month-old who presented after "accidental" cocaine intoxication.[49] All of these cases highlight the need to obtain a detailed history, to maintain a low level of suspicion for possible drug ingestion, even in the youngest patients, and to rule out administration of the drug by a caregiver. There are also a few case reports of accidental methamphetamine ingestion in the literature. One case series reviewed 47 cases of children under 6 years of age who had documented methamphetamine exposure.[50] In this series, the median age was 12 months. The most common symptom on presentation was agitation, which was present 82% of the time. Seizures, mild tachycardia, hypertension, and hyperpyrexia were also noted but less frequently. Another case report described an 11-month-old infant presenting to the emergency department after acute accidental intoxication from 3,4-methylenedioxymethamphetamine (MDMA, ecstasy).[51] This child presented with what was initially thought to be febrile seizures, depressed consciousness, repetitive and jerky movements of his limbs, hyperreflexia, muscle rigidity, dilated and unreactive pupils, perioral cyanosis, tachycardia, and hypertension. Urine toxicology screening was positive for MDMA and segmental hair analysis was positive for cocaine, indicating chronic exposure to this drug as well. Finally, there is a case report of two toddlers who tested positive for cocaine at the time of suffering first and second degree pharyngeal and esophageal burns after ingesting free-based cocaine, which can include alkaline caustics such as potassium hydroxide or ammonia.[52]

Cases of coma after ingestion of cannabis cookies have been reported,[53] indicating the importance of considering accidental ingestion in previously well children that present with unexplained coma. One of the affected children was an 11-month-old infant while another child demonstrated deep coma requiring airway support for partial obstruction. Other potential symptoms at presentation may be rapid onset of drowsiness, conjunctival hyperemia, papillary dilation, hyporeflexia, hypotonia, tachycardia, and presence of an oral residue, such as small granules or leaves.

It may be difficult to determine whether a child ingested an illegal substance accidentally or if it was given to the child by a caregiver for a particular effect. At least three cases in the literature tell of mothers giving their infants methadone to sedate them, leading in each case to the infant's death.[54,55] In all three cases, which involved a 14-month-old infant, a 5-month-old infant, and a 10-month-old infant, the mothers admitted to giving a small amount of the drug in an attempt to quiet their crying child. All three deaths were ruled homicides. There have also been reports of caregivers forcing ingestion of an illicit substance or alcohol for amusement of the caregiver or to produce a desired effect, such as quieting the child. One study showed 11% of adolescent females surveyed in one treatment program admitted to deliberately intoxicating children they were babysitting by blowing marijuana smoke in their faces.[56]

Passive exposure to illicit drugs may create risk for children. It remains unclear how much exposure causes a child to become symptomatic, but studies are examining that issue. One study is exploring the potential pulmonary irritant aspect of second-hand methamphetamine smoke by identifying lung injury in laboratory mice exposed to vaporized methamphetamine.[57] Although these studies are early and have not yet been translated to humans and children, they raise awareness of possible pulmonary risk to children living in these environments. Additionally, it has been shown that, after methamphetamine is smoked, methamphetamine residue contaminates surfaces at a level that may result in a positive drug test in a child living in that environment.[58] It is unclear if the exposure would be high enough to cause illness, but the evidence certainly raises concerns on yet another level for safety of children in these homes. Studies exploring similar risks of other smoked drugs have yet to be conducted. Such studies may be of some additional help in better understanding the risks of these environments.

Clandestine Methamphetamine Laboratories

Children in homes where methamphetamine is being manufactured represent another group at risk. Clandestine laboratories, most commonly used to manufacture methamphetamine, were once most commonly found in rural areas and on the West Coast as well as in the Midwest. Such laboratories are now appearing more often in urban and suburban areas. The laboratories use multiple hazardous chemicals, including acid and alkaline corrosives (eg, hydrochloric acid, sulfuric acid, sodium hydroxide or lye), anhydrous ammonia, lithium, red phosphorus, and solvents (eg, toluene, acetone, starting fluid, denatured alcohol) to convert pseudoephedrine or ephedrine to methamphetamine. Children are found in about 30% to 35% of these environments, which are extremely dangerous. The hazardous chemicals used in the manufacturing process are often improperly stored, such as in refrigerators and within reach of curious children. Numerous reports tell of children ingesting these dangerous chemicals, resulting in severe illness and death. One case report described the presentation of two children to the emergency department following severe caustic ingestions in homes where methamphetamine was being manufactured.[59] The first case involved a 5-year-old child who presented gasping and vomiting after ingesting a commercial cleaner containing sulfuric acid. The child required endotracheal intubation due to respiratory distress and suffered severe burns of the lips, tongue, oropharynx, and esophagus, as well as partial-thickness burns to the hands. The child ultimately required tracheostomy and gastrostomy tube placement and has subsequently required esophageal resection and replacement with a colonic conduit. In the second described case, a 2-year-old child was brought to the emergency department with drooling, stridor, and blistered skin of the neck, chest, and abdomen following ingestion of a substance containing sulfuric acid. He also required intubation and ultimately gastrostomy tube placement, as well as endoscopic esophageal dilation.

Many of these chemicals used to manufacture methamphetamine produce toxic vapors. Recent studies from National Jewish Hospital and Research Center indicate that these vapors (including hydrochloric acid, phosphine gas, anhydrous ammonia, and iodine) are released in potentially dangerous levels and also permeate every porous surface in the home.[60] These vapors also contain methamphetamine itself, which is deposited on every vertical and horizontal surface in the home. The manufacturing process requires combining these chemicals, often with the use of heat, creating an environment that is extremely flammable and explosive. The long-term implications of these chemical combinations are not known. Several pilot studies have shown that many of these children test positive for methamphetamine at the time of removal from the home containing the laboratory.

Neglect

In general, the use of illicit drugs and excessive amounts of alcohol poses many other risks for dependant children in the care of the user. While impaired, the caregiver is often unable to provide the consistent care, supervision, encouragement, and guidance that children need. The caregiver's obsession with using and manufacturing the drug may cause the them to neglect the child's medical and dental care. If intravenous routes are the preferred method of use, both loaded and used needles are often found laying out in the open and accessible to children. Additionally, some drugs may have unique features that place these children at additional risk. For example, because of the paranoid features of methamphetamine use, the caregivers almost always have weapons readily accessible in the home. They also frequently engage in violent behavior, such as domestic violence and child physical abuse. Methamphetamine considerably increases the sex drives of users, making them extremely hypersexual and often overly interested in pornography, including that of a very graphic nature. Therefore, a large amount of graphic pornographic material is frequently found in these homes. Children, in addition to being exposed to this material, may also be victimized themselves either because of poor supervision of the children around perpetrators or because of the hypersexualized behavior of a caregiver.

GENERAL MANAGEMENT OF THE DRUG-EXPOSED CHILD
History and Physical Examination

Whether the practitioner is caring for a newborn infant or an older child presenting to the office or emergency department, a detailed social history should be obtained as part of the routine medical evaluation. The history should include a nonjudgmental inquiry into drug and alcohol use in the home as well as the extent and context of the use. It is preferable to ask these questions with an affirmative approach (eg, "What drugs and alcohol are used in the home?" "By whom?" and "How much?") as this often creates an environment that elicits more honest, complete, and detailed information. This information may be critical to diagnosis and care of the child. It is also useful for identifying potential areas of need for support for the family. As the literature describing accidental and intentional ingestions of illegal drugs makes clear, it is important to obtain a detailed history that includes parents' therapeutic and recreational drug-use habits and to consider drug ingestions and exposures in children who present with an altered level of consciousness.

The physical examination of an infant or child potentially exposed to illegal drugs or alcohol is also important. For a newborn infant, in addition to the routine complete physical evaluation, special care should be taken to identify any features of FAS or early signs of withdrawal. For an older child, special attention should be paid to vital signs, especially for indications of catecholamine excess (such as hypertension, tachycardia, hyperpyrexia) or depression/sedation, as may be seen in opioid, marijuana, or alcohol ingestion. Additionally, assessment should include evaluation for signs of catecholamine depletion, such as lethargy. A complete head-to-toe examination is important to identify any signs or symptoms of physical or sexual abuse, including evaluation of the skin for burns. Laboratory work may be considered to assess for concomitant infection, anemia, electrolyte abnormality, and hypoglycemia.

Depending on the age of the child as well as the overall physical appearance, a head CT or skeletal survey may be considered. These children may have other signs and symptoms of abuse and neglect and the parental history may be incomplete and inaccurate.

Children removed from locations where methamphetamine (or other drugs) is being manufactured require some additional consideration because of the additional environmental and chemical hazards present. A medical protocol for such cases has been established through the efforts of a national group of clinicians, scientists, and researchers who assembled to formulate the best practice guidelines for children.[61] This document, available at the Web site of the National Alliance for Drug Endangered Children (www.nationaldec.org), provides color-coded pathways for the main disciplines responding to cases of this nature and includes recommendations for medical care. This group recommends that decontamination should be considered for a child removed from this environment once the child is deemed to be medically stable, especially if there has been indication of significant clinical exposure, such as an explosion or fire. If possible, the child's clothes should be removed and discarded and the child should be cleansed with a warm shower and soap when this can be done without additional trauma to the child. As soon as possible after the child's removal, the child's vital signs should be obtained and a full physical examination should be performed, paying particular attention to the neurologic and respiratory status. Because of the multiple pulmonary irritants found in these environments, any symptoms related to breathing, such as cough or wheezing, should be further assessed with a chest radiograph and further pulmonary evaluation.

Furthermore, a comprehensive history and physical evaluation should be undertaken within 72 hours after removal and a developmental screen should be performed as soon as feasible. Because of potential blood-borne pathogen exposures, additional laboratory assessment is suggested to assess for sexually transmitted diseases, such as HIV and hepatitis B and C. Other testing, such as chemistry profiles and blood counts, may be indicated based on clinical findings. Toxicology screening should be performed to identify any potential exposures, but urine catheterization should be avoided in an asymptomatic child. A medical home should be established for the child so that ongoing care and follow-up can be coordinated as needed.

Drug Testing

Testing can be useful to identify drug exposures in newborn infants and in older infants and children. Identifying pregnancies complicated by drug use is important for maternal, fetal, and newborn health. For all women at the time of delivery, clinicians should perform a thorough history that includes screening questions about prenatal drug and alcohol use. Meanwhile, defined criteria should be established for determining who should be tested for potentially exposing the fetus to drugs. Laboratory testing for drug use in pregnancy is a complex issue with medical, social, ethical, and legal implications. Testing may be a useful tool in determining whether or not an infant has been exposed. Then clinicians can formulate the most appropriate medical care plan, which may include monitoring for withdrawal symptoms and an early referral for developmental screening and intervention. However, for many reasons, tests may be negative for infants whose mothers used or abused drugs or alcohol. Criteria for testing should be largely based on medical factors known to be potentially related to drug exposure, such as unexplained placental abruption, maternal hypertension, precipitous delivery, intrauterine growth restriction/small for gestational age infant, premature rupture of membranes/labor/birth, microcephaly, signs/symptoms of drug withdrawal, and physical stigmata of FAS. Additionally, several social factors should be considered as reasons to test the infant at birth. These include mother's history of drug or excessive alcohol use as well as absent, late, or poor prenatal care. Depending on the hospital's policy, consent may need to be obtained prior to testing the mother or infant.

Methods of detection of prenatal drug and alcohol exposure have improved considerably in the past several years making testing quite reliable, accurate, and useable.[62] The matrices for testing have grown considerably and now include those from the fetus or newborn, such as meconium, fetal hair, cord blood and tissue, and neonatal urine; from the pregnant or nursing mother, such as hair, blood, oral fluid, sweat, urine, and breast milk; and from both the fetus and the mother, such as placenta and amniotic fluid.[63]

The primary historical method for testing newborn infants is through urine drug testing, although this may be challenging since the infant may urinate prior to being able to apply a urine collection bag and the bag does not always collect the urine adequately. Catheterization should not be undertaken unless there is an urgent medical indication. Additionally, because of metabolism rates of the drugs, detection of drugs in the urine is only helpful if the exposure occurred in the 3 to 7 days before testing.[64]

Another method of testing for prenatal drug exposure is the collection of meconium. Because this substance first forms in utero during the twelfth to thirteenth week of gestation and continues to accumulate during gestation, it serves as a reservoir for drugs and gives a much broader window of detection than other matrices.[24,65] Recent methods of testing meconium involve testing for fatty acid ethyl esters (FAEEs) as a biomarker for prenatal alcohol exposure.[66]

Hair testing has also become a promising method of detection of drugs and alcohol (through FAEEs) as it also provides for a long window of detection of months to years, making it a good method of testing for use during pregnancy.[24,66] Finally, recent work has shown promise in the use of umbilical cord tissue for the detection of longer-term fetal exposure to illegal drugs, such as methamphetamine, opiates, cocaine, and cannabinoids.[67,68]

Children presenting to medical care with otherwise unexplained symptoms, such as seizures, hypertension, tachycardia, and hyperpyrexia, as well as sedation or lethargy, should be evaluated for potential drug exposure or ingestion. Rapid urine toxicology may prevent unnecessary medical evaluation and treatments. Aspiration and analysis of gastric contents may be helpful in identifying the kind and level of drug ingestion. Additionally, serum can be held at the time of presentation for later testing as indicated.

Treatment

For an infant exposed to illegal drugs or alcohol prenatally, most treatment focuses on supportive care. For infants that display the signs and symptoms of neonatal abstinence syndrome related to sudden withdrawal of maternally transferred opioids, an optimal treatment has not been identified but specific opioid agents, such as morphine sulphate, neonatal opium solution or tincture of opium and methadone, have been used with some success.[69] One recent study has begun to explore the efficacy and safety of sublingually administered buprenorphine for the treatment of neonatal abstinence syndrome and has demonstrated an acceptable safety margin, although the safety and efficacy still needs to confirmed.[69]

For cases of accidental or intentional ingestion of drugs, careful attention should be given to the child's airway and breathing for any child presenting in an altered level of consciousness. Most treatment involves supportive care but in cases of deep coma, assisted ventilation may be required. Consultation with the local toxicology or poison center experts is encouraged. The use of benzodiazepines may be required to help control panic attacks in children who have ingested cannabinoids.[53] For a child presenting following ingestion of a stimulant, such as cocaine or amphetamines, supportive care is again the cornerstone of treatment. Benzodiazepines, such as diazepam, are the first line for pharmacologic intervention. In the most extreme situations, phenobarbital, pyridoxine, and paralysis with intubation may be required to treat/control seizures. Gastric lavage and administration of activated charcoal may be considered if very recent ingestion is suspected.

Finally, prevention through patient education is an essential consideration to reduce risks for children in homes where parents may be using illegal drugs or alcohol.

Reporting

Drug addiction is a serious and recurring disease. Ensuring the safety and well-being of children in environments with adults addicted to drugs is critical. Substance-abuse treatment is an important component in breaking the cycles of substance abuse and child abuse and neglect. However, because laws tend to emphasize punishment rather than treatment, the pregnant or parenting addict may not seek care, including prenatal care, for fear of revealing the addiction. Child protective services can be a partner with the medical care team in advocating for the families' needs and ensuring that the necessary services are available and used. Reporting laws require medical providers to report cases of suspected or known child abuse and neglect to child protective services. Many states now have laws requiring a report of an infant born exposed to or testing positive for illegal drugs. Additionally, child protection issues must be addressed in childhood poisonings whether they are thought to be accidental or intentional. A report to child protective services or law enforcement allows for a safety assessment of the home as well as a review and consideration of any potential history of previous child-welfare concerns with the family. Additionally, the report may trigger the provision of some necessary resources for the family.

Safety and support plans using foster homes, extended family, and community members, including the medical community, are essential to the continuing safety and well-being of the children and the continuing recovery of substance-abusing parents. However, studies of the families of substance-abusing mothers point out the vicious cycle of parents being neglected or abused as children and then perpetuating the neglect and abuse with their own children. Comprehensive programs that can identify the addicted parent, offer substance-abuse and addiction education and treatment, and provide necessary support services are most likely to meet the unique needs of substance-abusing mothers.

Substance-abuse treatment programs that are culturally responsive, immediately available, and include full wraparound services are the key to offering the parent the best chance at recovery and the child the best possible outcome. These services might include family group planning meetings with the extended family and community support providers, adequate housing, counseling for sexual and domestic violence, child care, health care (including family planning and well-child care, in addition to prenatal care), mental health care assistance, education, training, and employment. The child's regular medical provider may play an important role in supporting the family while continuing to direct the medical care for any of the child's identified needs.

Most drug-treatment programs have focused on males and not on the unique issues for women and their special needs during pregnancy and into the parenting years. Some of these issues include the need for child-care assistance, transportation, and job-skills training. Many of these women also need assistance with issues related to domestic violence, infectious diseases (such as HIV, hepatitis, tuberculosis), and mental health. More treatment programs where mothers reside with their children are needed. In addition, front-loading services and expanded family and community support can be effective for keeping children in the home while parents recover from substance abuse and simultaneous mental health problems, or receive other remedial or rehabilitative services.[70] Substance-abuse treatment must be a major component of the treatment plan for these families and needs to be made available in a timely manner. However, caregivers may fail to comply with drug and alcohol treatment programs within court-ordered guidelines. When that happens, early termination of parental rights should be considered so that the child can be placed in another, more stable living environment.

SUMMARY

Addressing the issues of substance abuse and child maltreatment is most effectively done through a multidisciplinary approach. The incorporation of the efforts of multiple disciplines, including those represented by the medical community, prevention services, law enforcement agencies, the courts, probation offices, child protective services, treatment centers, mental health services, educational organizations, federal agencies, nonprofit organizations, and the community, has emerged as the most promising approach to addressing this pervasive and challenging social problem. The National Alliance for Drug Endangered Children proposes that the solution to the problems of substance abuse and child maltreatment requires a focus on "the formation of community-based partnerships that encourage agency personnel from across these disciplines to coordinate mutual interests, resources and responsibilities." The involvement of the medical community in these efforts is critical to the identification and care of many of these at-risk children and to the success of these critical partnerships.

REFERENCES

1. U.S. Department of Health and Human Services, Substance Abuse and Mental Health Services Administration. 2007 National Survey on drug use and health: national findings. Rockville (MD): Substance Abuse and Mental Health Services Administration, Office of Applied Studies; 2008.
2. Child Welfare League of America & North American Commission on Chemical Dependency and Child Welfare. Children at the front; a different view of the war on alcohol and drugs. Washington, DC: Child Welfare League of America; 1992.
3. White WL, Illinois Department of Children and Family Services, Illinois Department of Alcoholism and Substance Abuse. SAFE 95: a status report on Project Safe, an innovative project designed to break the cycle of maternal substance abuse and child neglect/abuse. Springfield (IL): Illinois Department of Children and Family Services; 1995.
4. Kelleher K, Chaffin M, Hollenberg J, et al. Alcohol and drug disorders among physically abusive and neglectful parents in a community-based sample. Am J Public Health 1994;84:1586–90.
5. Health and Human Services, Public Health Service, Substance Abuse and Mental Health Services Administration & Office of Applied Studies. National household survey on drug abuse: main findings, 1996. Rockville (MD): Substance Abuse and Mental Health Services Administration, Office of Applied Studies; 1998.

6. Wang CT, Harding K. Current trends in child abuse reporting and fatalities: the results of the 1998 annual fifty state survey. Chicago: National Committee to Prevent Child Abuse; 1999.

7. Murphy JM, Jellinew M, Quinn D, et al. Substance abuse and serious child maltreatment: prevalence, risk, and outcome in a court sample. Child Abuse Negl 1991;15:197–211.

8. Reid J, Macchetto P, Foster S. No safe haven: children of substance-abusing parents. New York: National Center on Addiction and Substance Abuse at Columbia University; 1999.

9. Bays J. Substance abuse and child abuse–impact of addiction on the child. Pediatr Clin North Am 1990;37:881–904.

10. U.S. Department of Health and Human Services. Blending perspectives and building common ground: a report to congress on substance abuse and child protection. Washington DC: US Government Printing Office; 1999.

11. English DJ, Marshall DB, Brummel S, et al. Characteristics of repeated referrals to child protective services in Washington State. Child Maltreat 1999; 4(4):297–307.

12. Bennett EM, Kemper KJ. Is abuse during childhood a risk factor for developing substance abuse problems as an adult? J Dev Behav Pediatr 1994;15:426–9.

13. Kienberger Jaudes P, Ekwo E. Association of drug abuse and child abuse. Child Abuse Negl 1995;19(9):1065–75.

14. Finnegan LP. Perinatal morbidity and mortality in substance using families: effects and intervention strategies. Bull Narc 1994;46:19–43.

15. Finnegan LP, Kandall SR. Maternal and neonatal effects of alcohol and drugs. In: Lowinson JH, Ruiz P, Millman RB, et al, editors. Substance abuse—a comprehensive textbook. Section VII. Management of medical conditions associated with substance abuse. Baltimore (MD): Williams & Wilkins; 1997. p. 513–34.

16. Rivkin MJ, Davis PE, Lemaster JL, et al. Volumetric MRI study of brain in children with intrauterine exposure to cocaine, alcohol, tobacco, and marijuana. Pediatrics 2008;121(4):741–50.

17. Sayal K, Heron J, Golding J, et al. Prenatal alcohol exposure and gender differences in childhood mental health problems: a longitudinal population-based study. Pediatrics 2007;119:426–34.

18. Fried PA. Marihuana use by pregnant women and effects on offspring: an update. Neurobehav Toxicol Teratol 1982;4:451–4.

19. Lester B, Dreher M. Effects of marijuana use during pregnancy on newborn cry. Child Dev 1989;60:765–71.

20. Scher MS, Richardson GA, Coble PA, et al. The effects of prenatal alcohol and marijuana exposure: disturbances in neonatal sleep cycling and arousal. Pediatr Res 1988;24:101–5.

21. Carvalho de Moraes Barros M, Guinsburg R, Peres CDA, et al. Exposure to marijuana during pregnancy alters neurobehavior in the early neonatal period. J Pediatr 2006;149:781–7.

22. Fried PA, Watkinson B. 36- and 48-month neurobehavioral follow-up of children prenatally exposed to marijuana, cigarettes and alcohol. J Dev Behav Pediatr 1990;11(2):49–58.

23. American Academy of Pediatrics Committee on Drugs. Neonatal drug withdrawal. Pediatrics 1998;101:1079–88.

24. Huestis MA, Choo RE. Drug abuse's smallest victims: in utero drug exposure. Forensic Sci Int 2002;128:20–30.

25. Finnegan LP. Women, pregnancy and methadone. Heroin Add Rel Clin Probl 2000;2:1–8.
26. Lutiger B, Graham K, Einarson TR, et al. Relationship between gestational cocaine use and pregnancy outcome: a meta-analysis. Teratology 1991;44:405–14.
27. Richardson GA. Prenatal cocaine exposure. A longitudinal study of development. Ann N Y Acad Sci 1997;826:144–52.
28. Lewis BA, Kirchner L, Short EJ, et al. Prenatal cocaine and tobacco effects on children's language trajectories. Pediatrics 2007;120:e78–85.
29. Bada HS, Das A, Bauer SR, et al. Impact of prenatal cocaine exposure on child behavior problems through school age. Pediatrics 2007;119:348–59.
30. Arria AM, Derauf C, LaGasse LL, et al. Methamphetamine and other substance use during pregnancy: preliminary estimates from the Infant Development, Environment, and Lifestyle (IDEAL) study. Matern Child Health J 2006;10(3):293–302.
31. Smith LM, LaGasse LL, Derauf C, et al. The Infant Development, Environment, and Lifestyle Study: effects of prenatal methamphetamine exposure, polydrug exposure, and poverty on intrauterine growth. Pediatrics 2006;118:1149–56.
32. Kandall SR. Perinatal effects of cocaine and amphetamine use during pregnancy. Bull N Y Acad Med 1991;67:240–55.
33. Billing L, Eriksson M, Jonsson B, et al. The influence of environmental factors on behavioral problems in 8-year-old children exposed to amphetamine during fetal life. Child Abuse Negl 1994;18:3–9.
34. Weiner SM. Drug withdrawal in the neonate. In: Merenstein G, Gardner S, editors. Handbook of neonatal intensive care. St. Louis, (MO): Mosby-Year Book Inc.; 1998. p. 129–45.
35. Till C, Westall CA, Koren G, et al. Vision abnormalities in young children exposed prenatally to organic solvents. Neurotoxicology 2005;26:599–613.
36. Leventhal JM, Brown WC, Forsyth MB, et al. Maltreatment of children born to women who used cocaine during pregnancy: a population-based study. Pediatrics 1997;100(2):258 [abstract]. Available at: pediatrics.org/cgi/content/full/100/2/e7.
37. Chaney NE, Franke J, Waadlington WB. Cocaine convulsions in a breast-feeding baby. J Pediatr 1988;112:134–5.
38. Little RE, Anderson KW, Ervin CH, et al. Maternal alcohol use during breast-feeding and infant mental and motor development at one year. N Engl J Med 1989;321:425–30.
39. Chasnoff IF, Lewis DE, Squires L. Cocaine intoxication in a breast-fed infant. Pediatrics 1987;80:836–8.
40. JFL. Mother gets 6 years for drugs in breast milk [editorial]. Pediatrics 1994;93:103.
41. Bateman DA, Heargarty MC. Passive freebase cocaine ("crack") inhalation in infants and toddlers. Am J Dis Child 1989;143:25–7.
42. Heidemann SM, Goetting MG. Passive inhalation of cocaine by infants. Henry Ford Hosp Med J 1990;38:252–4.
43. Mirchandani HG, Mirchandani IH, Hellman F, et al. Passive inhalation of freebase cocaine ("crack") smoke by infants. Arch Pathol Lab Med 1991;115:494–8.
44. Bays J. Child abuse by poisoning. In: Reese RM, editor. Child abuse: medical diagnosis and management. Philadelphia: Lea & Febiger; 1994. p. 69–106.
45. Rosenberg NM, Meert KL, Knazik SR, et al. Occult cocaine exposure in children. Am J Dis Child 1991;145(12):1430–2.

46. Shannon M, Lacouture PG, Roa J, et al. Cocaine exposure among children seen at a pediatric hospital. Pediatrics 1989;83:337–41.
47. Lustbader AS, Mayes LC, McGee BA, et al. Incidence of passive exposure to crack/cocaine and clinical findings in infants seen in an outpatient service. Pediatrics 1998;103:e5.
48. Ernst AA, Sanders WM. Unexpected cocaine intoxication presenting as seizures in children. Ann Emerg Med 1989;18:774–7.
49. Garland JS, Smith DS, Rice TB, et al. Accidental cocaine intoxication in a nine-month old infant: presentation and treatment. Pediatr Emerg Care 1989;5(4): 245–7.
50. Matteucci MJ, Auten JD, Crowley B, et al. Methamphetamine exposures in young children. Pediatr Emerg Care 2007;23(9):638–40.
51. Garcia-Algar O, Lopez N, Bonet M, et al. 3,4-Methylenedioxymethamphetamine (MDMA) intoxication in an infant chronically exposed to cocaine. Ther Drug Monit 2005;27(4):409–11.
52. Massa N, Ludemann JP. Pediatric caustic ingestion and parental cocaine abuse. Int J Pediatr Otorhinolaryngol 2004;68:1513–7.
53. Appelboem A, Oades PJ. Coma due to cannabis toxicity in an infant. Eur J Emerg Med 2006;13:177–9.
54. Kintz P, Villain M, Dumestre-Toulet V, et al. Methadone as a chemical weapon—two fatal cases involving babies. Ther Drug Monit 2005;27(6):741–3.
55. Couper FJ, Chopra K, Pierre-Louis ML. Fatal methadone intoxication in an infant. Forensic Sci Int 2005;153:71–3.
56. Schwartz RH, Peary P, Mistretta D. Intoxication of young children with marijuana: a form of amusement for pot-smoking teenage girls. Am J Dis Child 1986;140: 326.
57. Wells SM, Buford MC, Braseth SN, et al. Acute inhalation exposure to vaporized methamphetamine causes lung injury in mice. Inhal Toxicol 2008;20(9): 829–38.
58. Martyny JW, Arbuckle SL, McCammon SC, et al. Methamphetamine contamination on environmental surfaces caused by simulated smoking of methamphetamine. J Chem Health Safety 2008;25–31.
59. Farst K, Duncan JM, Moss M, et al. Methamphetamine exposure presenting as caustic ingestions in children. Ann Emerg Med 2006;49(3):341–3.
60. Martyny JW, Arbuckly SL, McCammon CS Jr, et al. Chemical concentrations and contamination associated with clandestine methamphetamine laboratories. J Chem Safety 2007;10.1016/j.jchas.2007.01.012.
61. Grant P. Evaluation of children removed from a clandestine methamphetamine laboratory. J Emerg Nurs 2007;33(1):31–41.
62. Araojo R, McCune S, Feibus K. Substance abuse in pregnant women: making improved detection a good clinical outcome. Clin Pharmacol Ther 2008;83(4): 520–1.
63. Lozano J, Garcia-Algar O, Vall O, et al. Biological matrices for the evaluation of in utero exposure to drugs of abuse. Ther Drug Monit 2007;29(6): 711–34.
64. Halstead AC, Godolphin W, Lockitch G, et al. Timing of specimen collection is crucial and urine screening of drug dependent mothers and newborns. Clin Biochem 1988;21:59–61.
65. Wingert WE, Feldman MS, Kim MH, et al. A comparison of meconium, maternal urine and neonatal urine for detection of maternal drug use during pregnancy. J Forensic Sci 1994;39:150–8.

66. Koren G, Huston J, Gareri J. Novel methods for the detection of drug and alcohol exposure during pregnancy: implications for maternal and child health. Clin Pharmacol Ther 2008;83(4):631–4.
67. Montgomery DP, Plate C, Alder SC, et al. Testing for fetal exposure to illicit drugs using umbilical cord tissue vs. meconium. J Perinatol 2006;26:11–4.
68. Montgomery DP, Plate CA, Jones M, et al. Using umbilical cord tissue to detect fetal exposure to illicit drugs: a multicentered study in Utah and New Jersey. J Perinatol 2008;28:750–3.
69. Kraft WK, Gibson E, Dysart K, et al. Sublingual buprenorphine for treatment of neonatal abstinence syndrome: a randomized trial. Pediatrics 2008;122:e601–7.
70. Metsch LR, Rivers JE, Miller M, et al. Implementation of a family-centered treatment program for substance-abusing women and their children: barriers and resolutions. J Psychoactive Drugs 1995;27:73–83.

Tackling Child Neglect: A Role for Pediatricians

Howard Dubowitz, MD, MS[a,b,c],*

KEYWORDS

- Child neglect • Child maltreatment • Pediatrics
- Assessment • Management

WHY IS CHILD NEGLECT SO IMPORTANT?

Incidence/Prevalence

Neglect is by far the most common form of child maltreatment identified. In 2006, 64% of the 905,000 substantiated child protective services (CPS) reports were for neglect, 2.2% were for medical neglect, 16% were for physical abuse, 8.8% were for sexual abuse, and 6.6% were for psychological maltreatment.[1] Eight of 1000 children are identified as neglected, a rate that has been steady since the early 1990s. Medical personnel made 12% of the reports. Child neglect, however, often is not observed, detected, or reported to CPS,[2] and its true incidence probably is much higher.

A different approach to CPS reports was used in the Third National Incidence Study of Child Abuse and Neglect conducted in 1993 in 42 counties representative of the United States.[2] Community professionals, including pediatricians, were trained as "sentinels" to document instances meeting study definitions of child maltreatment, regardless of whether they were reported to CPS. Neglect was identified in 14.6 per 1000 children, with rates per 1000 of 4.9 for physical abuse and 2.1 for sexual abuse.

Data from other sources point to societal neglect—circumstances in which children's needs are not met largely because of inadequate services, policies, and programs. For example, children's mental health needs often are not met.[3] One study found that only 38% to 44% of children and youth meeting stringent criteria for a psychiatric diagnosis in the prior 6 months had had a mental health contact in the previous year.[4] Neglected dental care is widespread. A study of preschoolers found that 49% of 4-year-olds had cavities, and fewer than 10% were properly treated.[5]

This work was supported by Grant #90CA1749 from the U.S. Department of Health and Human Services, Administration on Children and Families.

[a] Department of Pediatrics, University of Maryland School of Medicine, 520 W. Lombard Street, 1st Floor, Baltimore, MD, USA

[b] Center for Families, University of Maryland, Baltimore, MD, USA

[c] Division of Child Protection, Department of Pediatrics, University of Maryland Hospital, Baltimore, MD, USA

* University of Maryland School of Medicine, 520 W. Lombard Street, 1st Floor, Baltimore, MD 21201.

E-mail address: hdubowitz@peds.umaryland.edu

Another study found that 8.6% of kindergarteners needed urgent dental care.[6] Neglected health care is common, and if access to health care and health insurance are regarded as basic needs in the United States, 8.7 million children (11.7%) experienced this form of neglect in 2006.[7]

Morbidity/Mortality

Neglect can have substantial and long-term effects on children's physical and mental health and on their psychosocial and cognitive development. A few illustrative examples are highlighted here; more information is available elsewhere.[8,9]

Physical effects

Inadequate food can lead to failure to thrive.[10] Inadequate health care can result in injuries not being treated,[11] health problems[8] and dental problems[5,6] not being identified or treated, or, in the extreme, death.[12] In 2006, it is estimated that 74% of fatalities resulting from child maltreatment involved neglect, including medical neglect in 1.9% of cases.[1] Most of these deaths resulted from inadequate supervision contributing to deaths by drowning or in fires.

Neuroimaging studies have shown the impact of neglect. Comparing different forms of maltreatment with controls, neglect was associated most strongly with smaller sizes of the corpus callosum.[13] Longitudinal research has found linkages between child neglect (as well as abuse and other adverse childhood experiences) and adult health decades later, such as an increased risk of liver disease[14] and ischemic heart disease.[15] A connection with asthma and lung cancer has been reported from the same Adverse Childhood Experiences study.[16]

Cognitive/academic effects

Neglected children perform worse academically than do non-neglected children, especially when neglect co-occurs with other forms of maltreatment.[17] Children who have a history of neglect have more school absences,[18] more retentions, and lower grades than non-neglected children.[17]

Psychosocial effects

Neglected children are more likely than non-neglected children to exhibit developmental, emotional, and behavioral problems.[19–21] At times neglected children are passive and withdrawn; at other times, they are aggressive.[22] Neglected children have fewer positive social interactions with peers than do non-neglected peers and often are less self-assured.[23] Adolescents without parents who provide both adequate supervision and nurturance may be at increased risk for behavior and emotional problems, such as engaging in high-risk behaviors. The Adverse Childhood Experiences study has shown increased risk for depression and suicidality decades later.[24] There also is added risk for involvement in the criminal justice system.[25]

Costs

The human costs associated with child neglect are enormous for the children, their families, the community, and society. A huge financial burden, conservatively estimated at 104 billion dollars annually, is associated with child maltreatment.[26]

Morality and Rights

In addition to the human and financial costs, there is a compelling moral argument for ensuring that children's needs are met adequately. Meeting children's needs also should be viewed as a human rights concern, as is well articulated in the United Nations Convention on the Rights of the Child.[27]

WHAT CONSTITUTES CHILD NEGLECT?

Defining child neglect is not an academic exercise. It guides the thinking about and the practices involved in identifying and approaching this prevalent problem. Clinicians often struggle with answering this question, especially in the context of state law and local CPS practice. State laws focus on omissions in care by parents or caregivers that result in actual or potential harm.[28] At least implicitly, parents are held responsible, or culpable, for failing to provide necessary care. Here is a frequent dilemma: is it reasonable and constructive to blame a parent for a lapse in care, such as not getting a prescription filled, especially when there are extenuating circumstances? Understandably, many pediatricians feel hesitant or uncomfortable invoking "neglect" and blaming parents. It therefore is useful to consider several factors that guide a conceptual definition of neglect as well as practice.

A view of Parental Responsibility and Blame

Parents are primarily responsible for meeting their children's needs. An ecological framework for understanding neglect, however, recognizes that there usually are multiple and interacting contributors to parenting, and to neglect. For example, a single mother who has lost her job and health insurance and is feeling depressed and stressed may not manage to buy the medicines for her daughter's asthma. Some situations are even further beyond parental control, such as inadequacies in a school system that fails to meet children's educational needs. That more than 9 million children are without health insurance also can be construed as a form of societal neglect. In general, CPS become involved only when the parental omission in care is the major contributor to the child's need(s) not being met, an issue that needs to be weighed in each individual situation.

An Alternative Definition of Neglect Centered on Children's Basic Needs (Rights)

An alternative is to view neglect as occurring when a child's basic needs are not met adequately, resulting in actual or potential harm.[29] This child-centered approach has several advantages. It fits well with a primary goal of pediatrics: helping ensure children's safety, health, and development. A child-centered definition is less blaming and more constructive, a key issue as pediatricians and others strive to work with families. It is helpful to be able to say, "This is why I'm worried about your child" rather than "Here's what you did wrong." This approach also draws attention to other contributors to neglect, in addition to parents, encouraging a broader response to underlying problems (ie, neglect is the symptom).

Clearly, not all circumstances within this broad view of children's unmet needs will meet criteria for CPS involvement; alternative interventions may be more appropriate. For example, a child may not receive medical treatment because the plan was not clearly communicated. It is possible to develop criteria for a subset of neglect circumstances where CPS involvement is appropriate.

How Much Care is Adequate? Neglect and a Continuum of Care

The extent to which a child's needs are met exists on a continuum from optimal to grossly inadequate, without natural cut points. A crude categorization of situations as "neglect" or "no neglect" often is simplistic. Seldom is a need met perfectly or not at all; cut-points usually are quite arbitrary. For example, it is difficult to determine at what point inadequate household sanitation is associated with harmful outcomes. With relatively few extreme situations, the gray zone is large. Even a relatively concrete area, such as the daily requirement for key nutrients, is not straightforward, and it is difficult to measure the extent to which these needs are met. Instead, crude estimates can be made. Examples of adequate health care include:

- Reasonable care is provided for minor problems (eg, cleaning a cut)
- Professional care is obtained for moderate to severe problems (eg, trouble breathing)
- Adequate treatment is obtained to optimize outcome and limit complications (ie, adherence to treatment regimen)
- The child receives recommended preventive health care (eg, immunizations)
- Professional care meets accepted health care standards (ie, appropriate treatment)

The last example illustrates again how deficits in care are not always caused by parents. Because the extent to which needs are met is on a continuum, one may categorize care, albeit crudely, as "excellent" (eg, the infant car-seat is always used), "adequate" (eg. The infant car-seat is usually used), or "inadequate" (eg, the car-seat is seldom used). Circumstances fitting in the middle of the continuum still should be addressed, even if they do not meet the threshold for neglect. Pediatricians' efforts to help ensure children's needs are met adequately or well are naturally not bound to a label of neglect.

The Quest for an Evidence-Based Definition of Neglect

Ideally, as clinicians strive to practice evidence-based medicine, a definition of neglect would be based on empiric data demonstrating the actual or probable harm associated with certain circumstances (eg, not receiving adequate emotional support). Although an evidence-based definition is a good goal, it is inherently difficult to achieve for most types of neglect.

Children's health, safety, and development occur within a complex ecology with multiple and interacting influences, making it difficult to discern the impact of a single risk factor, such as inadequate emotional support. The context of children's experiences also influences the likely impact of a given circumstance; a mature 9-year-old, for example, may do well alone at home for a few hours, whereas an unsupervised child with a fire-setting problem is a scary proposition. In some circumstances (eg, hunger, homelessness, abandonment), it probably is not necessary to have evidence documenting harm. It is abundantly clear that these conditions impair children's safety, health, and development.

Caution is needed not to assume that poor health outcomes are caused by inadequate care. The health problem (eg, brittle diabetes) may be inherently complex with a difficult course despite receiving and adhering to the recommended treatment. In practice, one must apply the best available knowledge to clarify whether a certain circumstance or pattern of experiences jeopardizes a child's well being. Situations in which the likelihood of harm is equivocal are best not considered as neglect, although here, too, efforts should be made to improve care. CPS generally become involved only when the care received is clearly inadequate.

Actual Versus Potential Harm

States' legal definitions of neglect generally include circumstances of potential harm; however, approximately one third of states restrict their practice to circumstances involving actual harm.[30] Potential harm is an important concern because the impact of neglect may be apparent only years later. In addition, the goal of prevention may be served by addressing neglect even if no harm is yet apparent.

It is often difficult, however, to predict the likelihood and nature of future harm. In some instances, epidemiologic data are useful. For example, one can estimate the increased risk of a serious head injury from a fall from a bicycle when a child is not wearing a helmet compared with that when the child's head is protected.[31] In contrast, predicting the likelihood of harm when an 8-year-old is left home alone for a few hours is difficult. Such circumstances often come to light only if actual harm ensues. Even when risks can be estimated, opinions may vary as to how seriously to weigh a risk. In addition to the likelihood of harm, the nature of the potential harm should be considered. Even a high likelihood of minor harm (eg, bruising from a short fall) might be acceptable. Life is not risk free. Indeed, children's development requires taking risks (eg, learning to walk and falling). In contrast, even a low likelihood of severe harm (eg, drowning) is not acceptable.

Neglect is a Heterogeneous Phenomenon

The different types of neglect children may experience represent a wide array of circumstances. This section briefly describes those most commonly encountered by pediatricians and makes specific suggestions for addressing them.

Non-adherence (noncompliance) with health care recommendations

Non-adherence is a form of neglect that occurs when recommendations for health care or further evaluation are not implemented, resulting in actual or potential harm. The term "non-adherence" is preferred because it avoids the blaming connotation of "noncompliance," recognizing the many potential contributors to health care recommendations not being implemented.[32] It is important to ascertain the extent to which treatment was not received and whether the child's problem is clearly attributable to inadequate care. Again, a child who has brittle diabetes might be out of control despite good care. It should be acknowledged that some recommended care might not be important (eg, a follow-up for an ear infection in an asymptomatic child); such lapses in care should not be labeled neglectful. Similarly, lapses in keeping primary care appointments for a healthy child are unlikely to result in harm and should not be considered neglect, although it is reasonable to encourage parents to adhere to the health maintenance schedule.

Identifying and addressing the barrier(s) to care is key, including careful consideration of the pediatrician–family relationship and the quality of communication. Management strategies also include clear communication, making the treatment as practical as possible, and follow-up to help ensure the plan is implemented successfully.

Delay or failure in receiving health care

Another form of medical neglect occurs when health care is needed but not obtained in a timely manner, or at all, resulting in actual or potential harm.[33] Parents or primary caregivers are responsible for recognizing health problems in their children and for taking care of minor needs, such as cleaning a cut. In more serious circumstances, they also are responsible for recognizing the need for professional care and helping the child obtain such care. They, in turn, need access to quality care.

CPS typically considers neglect when a child has a significant health problem that a parent or "average layperson" can reasonably be expected to respond to, but the caregiver fails to do so in a timely manner. For example, severe respiratory distress in a child who has asthma should be obvious; in contrast, asymptomatic lead poisoning is rarely apparent. In addition, there is a need to show that the lack of care harmed the child or jeopardized the child's health.

In assessing these situations, pediatricians should consider whether the delay in care was significant. For example, an infant may have had gastroenteritis for days but appear well, before abruptly decompensating with dehydration. Caution is needed before concluding, "If only the child had been brought in earlier, this ICU admission would have been avoided!"

As with other types of neglect, there may be multiple and interacting contributors to care not being obtained; understanding these factors is the guide to appropriate intervention. Failure or delay in receiving care may be related to maternal factors such as depression, to family factors such as a lack of transportation, and to community factors such as limited access to health care. Pediatricians may contribute unknowingly to medical neglect.[33] Parents often depend on pediatricians to explain a child's condition and plan for treatment. If the explanation is rushed or explained in "medicalese," parents may not understand the recommendations, resulting in errors and omissions in care. Pediatricians share in the responsibility to ensure that children receive adequate health care. Families and children who have chronic diseases need to be well educated regarding when to seek professional help.

Another circumstance involves different cultural practices, such as the Southeast Asian folkloric remedy of cao gio. Used for a variety of symptoms, cao gio involves vigorous rubbing of a hard object up and down the body. Bruising and welts commonly result. Aside from questions of abuse, concerns of neglect arise when alternative (to mainstream medicine) remedies are used and complications ensue, especially when effective medical treatment is available (eg, for bacterial meningitis). The appropriateness of intervening is guided by the level of certainty that the alternative approach is harmful and by whether a distinctly preferable treatment exists.[33]

Sensitivity and humility are essential in broaching cultural differences, and a satisfactory compromise should be sought.[34] Sensitive pediatricians avoid an ethnocentric approach (ie, believing one's own way is best). On the other hand, although it is important to respect different cultural practices, one must recognize that there are cultural practices that harm children (eg, female genital mutilation), and these practices should not be accepted. It may be best to intervene with family elders or leaders of the cultural group, encouraging them to modify their practice, minimizing the risk that a family deviating from their community norm will be ostracized.

The same principles apply in circumstances where children do not receive medical care for religious reasons. Thirty-nine states and the District of Columbia have religious exemptions in their civil codes on child abuse or neglect, exempting parents who do not provide or seek medical care for sick children, stating, for example, "that a child is not to be deemed abused or neglected merely because he or she is receiving treatment by spiritual means, through prayer according to the tenets of a recognized religion."[35] The American Academy of Pediatrics strongly opposes these exemptions, advocating that "the opportunity to grow and develop safe from physical harm with the protection of our society is a fundamental right of every child," and "the basic moral principles of justice and of protection of children as vulnerable citizens require that all parents and caretakers must be treated equally by the laws and regulations that have been enacted by state and federal governments to protect children."[35]

Working with parents and religious and cultural leaders and seeking a satisfactory compromise are important. Sometimes agreement cannot be reached, and the child is harmed or at risk of harm. Bross[36] presented criteria for legal involvement in this form of medical neglect. First, the treatment refused by the parents should have definite and substantial benefits over the alternative. Second, not receiving the recommended treatment should risk serious harm (death or severe impairment). Third, with treatment, the child is likely to enjoy a "high quality" life. Fourth, in the case of teenagers, the youth should consent to treatment. Ridgway[37] reviewed judicial opinions on 66 cases involving disputes between physicians and parents about the care of sick children. Physicians prevailed in 80% of disputes and in 90% of those that were religion-based.

Several studies in the United States have found considerable agreement regarding what constitutes child neglect among adults from different racial/ethnic and socioeconomic groups.[38] More broadly, the United Nations Convention on the Rights of the Child attests to a remarkable international consensus regarding what is needed to ensure children's health, development, and safety.[27]

Failure to thrive, overweight

It is important that the diagnosis of failure to thrive (FTT) be accurate, with a child's growth correctly plotted on an appropriate chart (eg, weight/age falling below the fifth percentile). The etiology of FTT often is multifactorial; the old dichotomy of "organic or nonorganic" is no longer recommended, because most growth problems involve both nutritional and psychosocial factors.[39] In that a child's basic nutritional needs are not adequately met, most children who have FTT can be said to experience neglect. CPS focuses on problems in which omissions in parental care are primarily responsible. It therefore is preferable to limit the label of neglect to such circumstances.

Pediatric overweight has increased dramatically in prevalence; more than 17% of children have a body mass index above the 95th percentile. There is continuity of overweight from preschool years through adulthood,[40] particularly when parents also are obese.[41] Morbidity associated with adult obesity includes cardiovascular problems, diabetes, psychosocial problems, and premature mortality. In a 10-year follow-up investigation of 1258 students (originally aged 9 to 10 years) in Copenhagen, Lissau and Sorensen[42] reported that, after controlling for age, demographics, and childhood body mass index, children who were neglected (received little parent support) were sevenfold more likely to become obese as young adults than children who were not neglected.

Like FTT, the etiology of overweight is invariably multifactorial, requiring a thorough assessment. Whatever the causes, neglect is a concern when serious growth problems are not being addressed despite access to appropriate services.

Drug-exposed newborns and older children

The compromised caregiving abilities of drug-abusing parents are a major concern. Parental substance abuse has been associated with child neglect.[43] Chaffin and colleagues[44] reported that approximately half the maltreating parents in their sample had a history of substance abuse and that drug abuse was associated with a threefold increase in child neglect. In addition, the potential harm to children of exposure to parental use of alcohol and other drugs has been shown.[45]

The pervasive use of legal but dangerous substances (ie, tobacco, alcohol) during pregnancy also raises an important issue, given present knowledge of the risks involved. It probably is not helpful to label any use of these substances as neglect; however, their use should be discouraged during pregnancy. The risk of second-hand smoke, especially to children who have pulmonary problems, is clear. The same principle applies: behaviors that counter children's basic needs and harm them constitute neglect. Approaches to prenatal drug exposure have varied greatly. Chasnoff and Lowder[46] offer an algorithm beginning with inducements to engage in drug treatment and leading to CPS and possible court involvement if therapeutic efforts fail.

Inadequate protection from environmental hazards

A basic need of children is to be protected from environmental hazards, inside and outside the home. Ingestions, injuries, exposure to guns, intimate partner violence, and failure to use car seats/belts may represent inadequate protection, threatening children's health. Through brief screening and anticipatory guidance, pediatricians can play important roles in helping parents recognize and prevent potential threats.[47] In general, a single incident (eg, ingestion) should not necessarily be seen as neglect, unless there is a pattern of inadequate supervision. Practical guidance on these issues is offered in the American Academy of Pediatrics The Injury Prevention Program and Violence Intervention and Protection Program resources.[48]

New and other forms of neglect

As knowledge evolves concerning children's health and development, new forms of neglect become apparent. For example, the impact of second-hand smoke on children, especially those who have pulmonary disease, has been recognized. Attitudes have shifted toward parents who leave guns accessible to children, sometimes resulting in tragic deaths. Approximately 15 states now have laws to hold these parents criminally liable, although only the Florida law has been found to reduce the rate of childhood deaths.[49] As it becomes increasingly common knowledge that infants should be placed on their backs to sleep, not doing so may, in the future, be perceived as a form of neglect.

Pediatricians may encounter several other forms of neglect, including inadequate nurturance and affection, abandonment, inadequate hygiene, inadequate clothing, and educational neglect. Information addressing such neglect is available in alternative resources.[8,9]

Other Aspects of Neglect that Influence the Response: Severity, Chronicity, Number of Incidents (Frequency), Intentionality, and the Context in which Neglect Occurs

Severity is viewed in terms of the likelihood and seriousness of harm. Simply put, severe neglect occurs when the unmet need is associated with serious harm, actual or potential. The greater the likelihood of harm, the more severe is the neglect.

Chronicity/frequency reflects a pattern of needs not being met. Some experiences are worrisome only when they occur repeatedly (eg, poor hygiene). Leaving an infant alone only once in a bathtub can have devastating results, however.

Intentionality regarding neglect is a question that arises, implicitly or explicitly. Intentionality probably does not apply to most neglectful situations. The *Merriam-Webster Dictionary* defines "intentional" as "done by intention or design." In most cases, parents do not intend to neglect their children's needs. Rather, problems impede their ability to meet these needs adequately. Even the most egregious cases, such as those in which parents seem willfully to deny their children food, probably involve significant psychopathology; labeling such instances "intentional" may be simplistic. In clinical practice, as pediatricians strive to strengthen families, viewing their shortcomings as intentional may be counterproductive, especially if doing so fosters a negative stance toward parents. As a practical matter, it is very difficult to assess intentionality.

Context is critical to thinking about neglect. For example, pediatricians may be understandably reluctant to consider the inability to fill a prescription because of a lack of funds as neglect. A mother who has no choice but to accept the night shift, resulting in her 10-year-old being in the apartment alone, poses a similar dilemma. Another example is a mother who resisted taking her child for therapy after his father had been killed despite the boy's depression several months later. She thought, "He'll be OK with time" and "Who's going to take him anyway? I need to work."

Such circumstances illustrate the complexity of neglect. It usually is not helpful to rush to judgment of these parents as neglectful. A constructive approach requires understanding the underlying circumstances to best tailor an approach that meets the needs of the individual child and family.

THE ETIOLOGY OF CHILD NEGLECT: A SYMPTOM WITH MANY POSSIBLE CONTRIBUTORS

Why are children neglected? Neglect is best understood as a symptom, with many possible contributors at the individual (parent and child), familial, community, and societal levels.[50] Professional actions and inactions also may contribute to neglect. Examples of each are highlighted briefly in the following sections. This ecological framework is critical for guiding a comprehensive assessment of what may be under-pinning the neglect, and an appropriate assessment should guide the intervention.

Parent

Mothers' mental health problems, especially depression and substance abuse, have been associated with neglect.[51,52] One study reported that whereas paternal absence alone was not associated with neglect, fathers or father figures who had been involved for a shorter period of time, who felt less efficacious in their parenting, and who were less involved in household tasks were more likely to have neglected children.[53] Another study found that children who described greater father support had a stronger sense of competence and social acceptance and fewer depressive symptoms.[54] When a child lacks a positive relationship with his or her father, this lack can be seen as a form of, or as a contributor to, neglect.

Child

Child characteristics such as low birth weight or prematurity may contribute to neglect.[55] Some studies have found increased maltreatment among children who have chronic disabilities.[56] In a more recent study, children who have mental health problems were at higher risk for maltreatment, but those who had developmental disabilities were not.[57]

Family

Intimate partner violence and child maltreatment frequently co-occur;[58] it is estimated that 50%[59] to 77%[60] of children exposed to intimate partner violence are maltreated also.

Community

The community context and its resources influence parent–child relationships and possible maltreatment. Parents' negative perceptions of the quality of neighborhood life have been found to be related to maltreatment.[61]

Society

Many factors at the broader societal level may compromise parents' abilities to care adequately for their children. In addition, these societal or institutional problems can be directly neglectful of children. In a national study, only 70% of children who had learning disabilities received special education services according to their parents; fewer than 20% of children receive needed mental health care.[62] Poverty seems to be strongly associated with neglect: "these families are the poorest of the poor."[63]

The harmful effects of poverty on the health and development of children are clear. In addition to its influence on family functioning, poverty directly threatens and harms children's health, development, and safety.[64] Although poverty correlates strongly with neglect, most children in low-income families are not neglected by their families. Nor are middle-class families immune to neglect.

Professionals

Professionals also may contribute to neglect. Problematic communication resulting in parents not understanding their child's condition or treatment plan is pervasive.[65] Pediatricians may not comply with recommended approaches, compromising children's health.[66] Pediatricians may fail to identify children's medical or psychosocial needs, contributing to neglect.

GENERAL PRINCIPLES FOR ASSESSING POSSIBLE NEGLECT

The heterogeneity of neglect precludes specific details for assessing the array of possible circumstances. Instead, the following general principles and questions help guide the assessment.

- Given the complexity and possible ramifications of determining whether a child is being neglected, an interdisciplinary assessment is ideal, including input from professionals involved with the family.
- Verbal children should be interviewed separately, at an appropriate developmental level. Possible questions include "Who do you go to if you're feeling sad?," "Who helps you if you have a problem?," and "What happens when you feel sick?"
- Do the circumstances indicate that the child's needs are not being adequately met? Is there evidence of actual harm? Is there evidence of potential harm and on what basis?
- What is the nature of the neglect?
- Is there a pattern of neglect? Are there indications of other forms of neglect, or abuse? Has there been prior CPS involvement?
- A child's safety is a paramount concern. What is the risk of imminent harm, and of what severity?
- What factors are contributing to the neglect? Consider the factors listed in the section "Etiology."
- What strengths/resources are there? Identifying these factors is as important as identifying problems.
  - Child (eg, child wants to play sports, requiring better health)
  - Parent (eg, parent wants to keep child out of the hospital)
  - Family (eg, other family members willing to help)
  - Community (eg, programs for parents, families)
- What interventions have been tried, with what results? Knowing the nature of the interventions can be useful, including from the parent's perspective. What has the pediatrician done to address the problem?
- Assess the possibility of other children in the household also being neglected, a common occurrence.[67]
- What is the prognosis? Is the family motivated to improve the circumstances and accept help, or resistant? Are suitable resources, formal and informal, available?

GENERAL PRINCIPLES FOR ADDRESSING CHILD NEGLECT

The following practices help in addressing cases of child neglect.

- Convey concerns to family, kindly but forthrightly. Avoid blaming.
- Be empathic and state interest in helping or suggest another pediatrician.
- Address contributory factors, prioritizing those most important and amenable to being remedied (eg, recommending treatment for a mother's depression). Parents' problems may need to be addressed to enable them to care for their children adequately. Parent training programs can be helpful.[68]
- Begin with least intrusive approach, usually not CPS.
- Establish specific objectives (eg, diabetes will be adequately controlled), with measurable outcomes (eg, urine dipsticks, hemoglobin A1c). Similarly, advice should be specific and limited to a few reasonable steps. A written contract can be very helpful, with one copy for the parent and one for the medical chart.
- Engage the family in developing the plan; solicit their input and agreement.
- Build on strengths; there always are some, providing a valuable hook to engage parents who may be reluctant to do so.
- Encourage positive family functioning. Videka-Sherman[69] described the need to focus on building positive family experiences, "not just controlling or decreasing negative interaction."
- Be innovative and consider resources, such as using pots and pans for play. Encouraging reading can promote both literacy and intimacy.[70]
- Encourage informal supports (ie, family, friends; encourage fathers to participate in office visits). Most people get most of their support from family and friends, not from professionals.
- Consider support available through a family's religious affiliation.
- Consider need for concrete services (eg, Medical Assistance, Temporary Assistance to Needy Families, food stamps).
- Consider children's specific needs, given what is known about the possible outcomes of neglect. Too often, maltreated children do not receive direct services.
- Be knowledgeable about community resources and facilitate appropriate referrals.
- Consider the need to involve CPS, particularly when moderate or serious harm is involved and when less intrusive interventions have failed. Present the report as a necessary effort to clarify what is occurring and what might be needed to help the child and family. In recent years a majority of states have developed an alternative response system, especially for neglect. This approach focuses primarily on supporting families to do better rather than on investigating what was done. It attempts to be conciliatory and constructive, rather than punitive. Most importantly, it prioritizes the crux of the issue: addressing the needs of children and families.
- Provide support and follow-up, review progress, and adjust the plan if needed.
- Recognize that neglect often requires long-term intervention with ongoing support and monitoring.
- Try to ensure continuity of care as the primary health care provider.

PREVENTING CHILD NEGLECT: A ROLE FOR PEDIATRICIANS

Instead of addressing the consequences of child neglect, it would be far preferable to help prevent the problem. There are several ways that pediatricians can do so. In addition to helping prevent child neglect and abuse, these strategies can enhance family functioning, support parents, and help ensure children's health, development, and safety.

The social history offers an opportunity to learn what is happening within the family, and there are brief questionnaires that can screen for specific problems, such as depression, intimate partner violence, and substance abuse.[71–73] Often these problems are well masked and go undetected. Ideally, screens should be applied universally within the practice. The Safe Environment for Every Kid model offers a promising approach.[74]

Astute observation is a critical tool, noting the appearance and behavior of parent(s) and child and their interactions. In addition to noting problems (eg, the parent appears to be high on drugs), efforts should be made to identify strengths.

For children who have chronic diseases, health education and extra support help ensure adequate care. Anticipatory guidance aims to ensure children's safety and well being. Pediatricians' support, monitoring, and counseling are useful ways to help families take adequate care of their children. Encouraging fathers to come in for routine visits and engaging them may help encourage increased involvement in their children's lives. At times, referrals to other professionals and agencies are necessary; helping a family obtain appropriate services is another valuable role that pediatricians play.

PRINCIPLES OF CHILD AND FAMILY ADVOCACY

As noted earlier, problems at several levels can contribute to child neglect. Pediatricians can be effective advocates on behalf of children and families in several ways. Explaining to a parent the safety needs of an increasingly mobile and curious toddler is one form of advocacy. Helping a family obtain services is another form of advocacy, as is remaining involved after a CPS report. Efforts to develop programs in a community and to improve policies and institutional practices concerning children and families also are important forms of advocacy. At the broader level of state and national government, pediatricians can advocate for policies and resources to help meet the needs (rights) of children and families. This advocacy role fits well with the mission of pediatrics, and it is much needed.

REFERENCES

1. U.S. Department of Health and Human Services. Administration on Children Youth and Families. Child maltreatment 2006. Washington (DC): U.S. Government Printing Office; 2008.
2. Sedlack AJ, Broadhurst DD. Third National Incidence Study of Child Abuse and Neglect: final report. Washington (DC): U.S. Department of Health and Human Services; 1996.
3. U.S. Department of Health and Human Services. Mental health: a Report of the Surgeon General—executive summary. Substance Abuse and Mental Health Services Administration, Center for Mental Health Services, National Institutes of Health, National Institute of Mental Health. Rockville (MD): U.S. Department of Health and Human Services; 1999.
4. Leaf P, Alegria M, Cohen P, et al. Mental health service use in the community and schools: results from the four-community MACA study. J Am Acad Child Adolesc Psychiatry 1996;35:889–97.
5. Tang J, Altman D, Robertson D, et al. Dental caries: prevalence and treatment levels in Arizona preschool children. Public Health Rep 1997;112:319–31.

6. Chung LH, Shain SG, Stephen SM, et al. Oral health status of San Francisco public school kindergarteners 2000-2005. J Public Health Dent 2006;66(4):235–41.
7. Cover The Uninsured. Available at: www.covertheuninsured.org. Accessed September 19, 2008.
8. Dubowitz H, Giardino A, Gustavson E. Child neglect: a concern for pediatricians. Pediatr Rev 2000;21(4):111–6.
9. Dubowitz H, Black M. Child neglect. In: Reece R, Christian C, editors. Child abuse: medical diagnosis and management. 3rd edition. Elk Grove Village (IL): American Academy of Pediatrics; 2008.
10. Krugman SD, Dubowitz H. Failure to thrive. Am Fam Physician 2003;68:879–84.
11. Overpeck MD, Kotch JB. The effect of US children's access to care on medical attention for injuries. AM J Public Health 1995;85:402–4.
12. Dubowitz H. Fatal child neglect. In: Alexander R, editor. Child fatality review. St. Louis (MO): G.W. Publishers; 2007.
13. Teicher MH, Dumont NL, Ito Y, et al. Childhood neglect is associated with reduced corpus callosum area. Biol Psychol 2004;56:80–5.
14. Dong M, Dube SR, Felitti VJ, et al. Adverse childhood experiences and self-reported liver disease: new insights into a causal pathway. Arch Intern Med 2003;163:1949–56.
15. Dong M, Giles WH, Felitti VJ, et al. Insights into causal pathways for ischemic heart disease: adverse childhood experiences study. Circulation 2004;110:1761–6.
16. Brown DW, Young KE, Anda RF, et al. Asthma and the risk of lung cancer. Findings from the adverse childhood experiences (ACE). Cancer Causes Control 2006;17(3):349–50.
17. Eckenrode J, Kendall-Tackett KA. School performance and disciplinary problems among abused and neglected children. Child Abuse Negl 1996;20(3):161–9.
18. Wodarski JS, Kurtz PD, Gaudin JM, et al. Maltreatment and the school-age child: major academic, socioemotional, and adaptive outcomes. Soc Work 1990;35:506–13.
19. Dietrich KN, Starr RH, Weisfeld OE. Infant maltreatment: caretaker-infant interaction and developmental consequences at different levels of parenting failure. Pediatrics 1983;72:332–40.
20. Aragona JA, Eyberg SM. Neglected children: mothers' report of child behavior problems and observed verbal behavior. Child Dev 1981;52:596–602.
21. Dubowitz H, Papas MA, Black MM, et al. Child neglect: outcomes in high-risk urban preschoolers. Pediatrics 2002;109(6):1100–7.
22. Bousha DM, Twentyman CT. Mother-child interactional style in abuse, neglect, and control groups: naturalistic observations in the home. J Abnorm Psychol 1984;93:106–14.
23. Hoffman-Plotkin D, Twentyman CT. A multimode assessment of behavioral and cognitive deficits in abused and neglected preschoolers. Child Dev 1984;55:794–802.
24. Dube SR, Anda RF, Felitti VJ, et al. Childhood abuse, household dysfunction, and the risk of attempted suicide throughout the life span: findings from the adverse childhood experiences study. JAMA 2001;286(24):3089–96.
25. Widom CS. The cycle of violence. Science 1989;244(4901):160–6.
26. Prevent Child Abuse America. Available at: http://member.preventchildabuse.org/site/DocServer/cost. Accessed November 20, 2008.
27. UNICEF. Convention on the Rights of the Child. Available at: http://www.unicef.org/magic/briefing/uncorc.html. Accessed November 30, 2008.
28. DePanfilis D. How do I determine if a child is neglected?. In: Dubowitz H, DePanfilis D, editors. Handbook for child protection practice. Thousand Oaks (CA): Sage; 2007. p. 121–6.

29. Dubowitz H, Black M, Starr R, et al. A conceptual definition of child neglect. Crim Justice Behav 1993;20:8–26.
30. Zuravin SJ. Issues pertinent to defining child neglect. In: Morton TD, Salovitz B, editors. The CPS response to child neglect: an administrator's guide to theory, policy, program design and case practice. Georgia: National Resource Center on Child Maltreatment; 2001. p. 1–22.
31. Wesson D, Spence L, Hu X, et al. Trends in bicycling-related head injuries in children after implementation of a community-based bike helmet campaign. J Pediatr Surg 2000;35(5):688–9.
32. Liptak GS. Enhancing patient compliance in pediatrics. Pediatr Rev 1996;17: 128–34.
33. Dubowitz H. Neglect of children's health care. In: Dubowitz H, editor. Neglected children: research, practice and policy. Thousand Oaks (CA): Sage Publications; 1999. p. 109–31.
34. Korbin J, Spilsbury J. Cultural competence and child neglect. In: Dubowitz H, editor. Neglected children: research, practice and policy. Thousand Oaks (CA): Sage Publications; 1999. p. 69–88.
35. American Academy of Pediatrics. Committee on Bioethics. Religious objections to medical care. Pediatrics 1997;99:279–81.
36. Bross DC. Medical care neglect. Child Abuse Negl 1982;6:375–81.
37. Ridgway D. Court-mediated disputes between physicians and families over the medical care of children. Arch Pediatr Adolesc Med 2004;158(9):891–6.
38. Dubowitz H, Klockner A, Starr R, et al. Community and professional definitions of neglect. Child Maltreat 1998;3:235–43.
39. Frank DA, Blenner S, Wilbur MB, et al. Failure to thrive. In: Reece RM, Christian C, editors. Child abuse: medical diagnosis and management. 3rd edition. Elk Grove Village (IL): American Academy of Pediatrics; 2009. p. 465–511.
40. Serdula MK, Ivery D, Coates RJ, et al. Do obese children become obese adults? A review of the literature. Prev Med 1993;22:167–77.
41. Whitaker RC, Wright JA, Pepe MS, et al. Predicting obesity in young adulthood from childhood and parental obesity. N Engl J Med 1997;337:869–73.
42. Lissau I, Sorensen TI. Parental neglect during childhood and increased risk of obesity in young adulthood. Lancet 1994;343:324–7.
43. Ondersma SJ. Predictors of neglect within low socioeconomic status families: the importance of substance abuse. Am J Orthop 2002;72:383–91.
44. Chaffin M, Kelleher K, Hollenberg J. Onset of physical abuse and neglect: psychiatric, substance abuse and social risk factors from prospective community data. Child Abuse Negl 1996;20:191–200.
45. Besinger BA, Garland AF, Litrownik AJ, et al. Caregiver substance abuse among maltreated children placed in out-of-home care. Child Welfare 1999;78:221–39.
46. Chasnoff IJ, Lowder LA. Prenatal alcohol and drug use and risk for child maltreatment: a timely approach to intervention. In: Dubowitz H, editor. Neglected children: research, practice and policy. Thousand Oaks (CA): Sage Publications; 1999. p. 132–55.
47. Dubowitz H, Prescott L, Feigelman S, et al. Screening for intimate partner violence in an urban pediatric primary care clinic. Pediatrics 2008;121(1):85–91.
48. American Academy of Pediatrics. Available at: http://www.aap.org. Accessed December 1, 2008.
49. Webster D, Starnes M. Reexamining the association between child access prevention gun laws and unintentional shooting deaths of children. Pediatrics 2000;106(6):1466–9.

50. Belsky J. Child maltreatment: an ecological integration. Am Psychol 1980;35: 320–35.
51. Polansky N, Chalmers M, Williams DP, et al. Damaged parents: an anatomy of child neglect. Chicago: University of Chicago; 1981.
52. Hoffman C, Crnic KA, Baker JK. Maternal depression and parenting: implications for children's emergent emotion regulation and behavioral functioning. Parenting Sci Pract 2006;6:271–95.
53. Dubowitz H, Black MM, Kerr M, et al. Fathers and child neglect. Arch Pediatr Adolesc Med 2000;154:135–41.
54. Dubowitz H, Kerr M, Cox C, et al. Father involvement and children's functioning at age 6: a multi-site study. Child Maltreat 2001;6(4):300–9.
55. Benedict M, White RB. Selected perinatal factors and child abuse. Am J Public Health 1985;75:780–1.
56. Benedict MI, White RB, Wulff LM, et al. Reported maltreatment in children with multiple disabilities. Child Abuse Negl 1990;14:207–17.
57. Jaudes PK, Mackey-Bilaver L. Do chronic conditions increase young children's risk of being maltreated? Child Abuse Negl 2008;32(7):671–81.
58. Hazen AL, Connelly CD, Kelleher K, et al. Intimate partner violence among female caregivers of children reported for child maltreatment. Child Abuse Negl 2004;28: 301–19.
59. Straus MA, Gelles RJ, Smith C. Physical violence in American families: risk factors and adaptations to violence in 8145 families. New Brunswick (NJ): Transactions Publishers; 1989.
60. American Academy of Pediatrics policy statement. The role of the health professional in recognizing and intervening on behalf of abused women. Pediatrics 1998;101:1091–2.
61. Garbarino J, Sherman D. High-risk neighborhoods and high-risk families: the human ecology of child maltreatment. Child Dev 1980;51:188–98.
62. Burns BJ, Costello EJ, Angold A, et al. Children's mental health service use across service sectors. Health Aff 1995;14:147–59.
63. Giovannoni JM, Billingsley A. Child neglect among the poor: a study of parental adequacy in families of three ethnic groups. Child Welfare 1970;84:196–214.
64. NICHD. Duration and developmental timing of poverty and children's cognitive and social development. Child Dev 2005;76:795–810.
65. Farrell MH, Kuruvilla P. Assessment of parental understanding by pediatric residents during counseling after newborn genetic screening. Arch Pediatr Adolesc Med 2008;162(3):199–204.
66. Lam BC, Lee J, Lau YL. Hand hygiene practices in a neonatal intensive care unit: a multimodal intervention and impact on nosocomial infection. Pediatrics 2004; 114(5):e565–71.
67. Hines DA, Kantor GK, Holt MK. Similarities in siblings' experiences of neglectful parenting behaviors. Child Abuse Negl 2006;30(6):619–37.
68. Edwards A, Lutzker JR. Iterations of the safe care model: an evidence-based child maltreatment prevention program. Behav Modif 2008;32(5):736–56.
69. Videka-Sherman L. Intervention for child neglect: the empirical knowledge base. In: Cowan A, editor. Current research on child neglect. Rockville (MD): Aspen Systems Corporation; 1988.
70. Duursma E, Augustyn M, Zuckerman B. Reading aloud to children: the evidence. Arch Dis Child 2008;93(7):554–7.
71. Lane W, Dubowitz H, Feigelman S, et al. Screening for parental substance abuse in an urban Pediatric primary care clinic. Ambul Pediatr 2007;7:458–62.

72. Dubowitz H, Feigelman S, Lane W, et al. Screening for depression in an urban pediatric primary care clinic. Pediatrics 2007;119(3):435–43.
73. Dubowitz H, Feigelman S, Lane W, et al. Pediatric primary care to help prevent child maltreatment: the Safe Environment for Every Kid (SEEK) model. Pediatrics, in press.
74. Dubowitz H. Preventing child neglect and physical abuse: a role for pediatricians. Pediatr Rev 2002;23(6):191–6.

Child Fatality Review Teams

Michael Durfee, MD[a],*, Juan M. Parra, MD, MPH[a],
Randell Alexander, MD, PhD[b]

KEYWORDS

• Child abuse • Death • Fatality review

The history of child fatality review (CFR) begins with the work of Ambrose Tardieu in 1860. More than a century later, in 1978, the first team was established in Los Angeles, California. This article reviews the history of CFR, the composition of teams, and its purpose based in preventive public health. The successes of 3 decades and challenges for the future of CFR are discussed.

OVERVIEW

French Physician Ambrose Tardieu described fatal child abuse in detail in 1860.[1] Dr Tardieu wrote in ornate French detailing the injuries of dead children. He added comments about the skepticism of his colleagues, who apparently ignored his work. Child abuse, however, was not widely acknowledged for a century, until the publication of "The Battered Child Syndrome" by C. Henry Kempe, MD and colleagues in the *Journal of the American Medical Association* in 1962.[2] This publication led to the development of laws requiring the reporting of child abuse in all 50 states. Child protective services assumed a more substantial role in the early 1970s with the passage of the Child Abuse Prevention and Treatment Act (PL 93-274) by Congress, and increased law enforcement and prosecution followed shortly thereafter. Child abuse was not indexed in the medical literature (Index Medicus) until 1965, and the topic of infanticide was not added until 1970.

Major response to fatal child abuse grew in the late 1980s and the 1990s with expansion of state child death review teams. A diverse group of professionals created the early child death review teams, building on other multiagency programs that were developing in child abuse assessment and prevention programs. Social changes after World War II may be part of the reason that such programs became possible. These changes included the expanding roles for women, which may have been a necessary

[a] Department of General Pediatrics, University of Texas Health Science Center at San Antonio Medical School, 7703 Floyd Curl Dr. Mail Code 7808, San Antonio, TX 78229-3900, USA
[b] Department of Pediatrics, Division of Child Protection and Forensic Pediatrics, University of Florida–Jacksonville, 4539 Beach Boulevard, Jacksonville, FL 32207, USA
* Corresponding author.
E-mail address: michaeld65@mac.com (M. Durfee).

Pediatr Clin N Am 56 (2009) 379–387
doi:10.1016/j.pcl.2009.01.004
0031-3955/09/$ – see front matter

precursor to the increased social status of children, professional and public acceptance that child abuse does occur, and the understanding that child abuse is a public health issue. Team members were exposed to child death, particularly deaths of infants and toddlers. They met counterparts from other professions and learned the value of multiagency team case management. New skills and relationships developed that were helpful in the review of nonfatal cases and in the development of prevention programs. This article discusses the change in the response of professionals to fatal child abuse from Dr. Tardieu's time to the present.

EARLY INFORMAL PEER SUPPORT

In the history CFR, it is clear that the motivation, skills, and leadership of early advocates led to the successful national and international expansion of both the purpose and scope of CFR. Child deaths are painful both to line professionals and to local people who have seen, heard, and touched the child who died. Being close to a child during his life makes the death more of a loss. Team dedication often was driven in part by the pain that accompanies the death of a child. Thus many teams found direction and informal support from members of other teams.

Some teams formed in response to a notorious child abuse fatality. Early case intake and review was expanded beyond abuse to include all injury deaths. Most early, informal teams were local and consisted of members who were on or near the front line of community interaction in their profession. The organizer's task required calling multiple agencies, arranging a room, creating and sharing a list of cases, and being positive. Social skills and tenacity were critical. Maternal mortality review, which measured the death of mothers in childbirth with reports originating in New Jersey in 1938, may have been the first ongoing death review in the United States.

FORMAL TEAMS

The first CFR team began in 1978 in Los Angeles County and was housed in the Interagency Council on Child Abuse and Neglect (ICAN), which had multiagency groups working in other areas.[3] Some questioned the benefits of discussing dead children. A few stated their lack of interest, but those who were invited came to the review. The value of child death review was understood after the first case reviews, as members discovered that each member was lacking information that others could provide. The story of the death became more complete and more real. Case management improved with more complete and more competent information of the events leading to death. A few cases with suspicious injuries were explained reasonably and labeled accidental deaths. Some other reviews uncovered a hidden or incomplete homicide investigation.

San Diego County created the second team in 1982. In contrast to the Los Angeles County cases, which showed a peak for fatal child abuse in the first year of life, the San Diego team initially found a peak for fatal child abuse at age 3 years. The San Diego team increased its focus on infants after consultation with the Los Angeles County team resulted in modifications of their Dan Diego case intake process and yielded an increase in missed suspicious infant deaths. Formal data collection and analysis reaffirmed some early premises, including the fact that infants comprise about 40% of the total cases of fatal child abuse. National data from the US Department of Health and Human Services (USDHHS) confirm these data today.[4]

About a dozen California counties had similar review teams by the mid 1980s, when Oregon, South Carolina, and Missouri initiated teams. Oregon used the California experience to build the first state team with logical structures that provided a model for other states. British Columbia, Canada, and New South Wales, Australia led international expansion with team reports in 1994. ICAN was appointed the National Center on Child Fatality Review with funds from US Department of Justice and endorsement from USDHHS. In 2000, all but one state had CFR teams, surpassing the US Surgeon General's objective of 44 states with CFR. The final state was added in 2001 by legislation.

Individuals from multiple professions took the lead to form CFR teams in the late 1970s and into the 1980s. Most of these pioneers were women. Early teams built from the bottom up rather than from the top down. Many early teams lacked authority and funding. Many early advocates of CFR simply contributed additional time to make the team a reality. They often avoided official governmental mandates, funding, and legal opinions, which could provide resources eventually but required time and could hinder the process. Such official actions came later, after multiple states had teams. Organizers needed few resources. The peer group supplied the skills, and the individual case provided the motivation.

Teams built from the top down, through legislation or executive order, occurred later, with both positive and negative results. Some legislation protected team confidentiality and encouraged members to share all information, including agency failures in case management. Other laws or mandates denied teams the opportunity to improve local team decisions by defining who would be the local chair or which cases could be reviewed, often limiting access to cases with previous Child Protection Services (CPS) records. Agency investigation of previous case management decisions after a death is necessary but can generate stress for the agency and the individuals involved in case. Case managers may be blamed or blame themselves for a death. Participation in group review identifies competence in case management rather than assigning blame. Guilt and shame after a child's death can last a lifetime, and participation in the response to the death can lessen that pain. Anxiety related to a group's review of a death may be tempered by having a supervisor or other frontline staff attend the review.

The multiagency team approach helped professionals from different disciplines create alliances that assisted with case management in future cases. Some team members discovered common issues, as well as differences, across professions with their location of work and knowledge of neighborhoods and even common families. Public health nurses, law enforcement, fire, and emergency rescue workers, coroner investigators, and CPS workers all work in potentially hazardous neighborhoods and homes, whereas others work safely in offices. Line-staff case managers learned the benefit that could be gained through the insight from other professions and the potential benefit of sharing records that previously had been separate. Prosecutors learned to support child witnesses and advocated for prevention programs. Human service professionals learned the potential benefits of involving the criminal justice system.

The teams that began with a focus on child abuse fatality rapidly expanded to include other deaths. Case reviews identified system failures and often led to prevention programs addressing other preventable causes of death, such as suicide, pool safety, safe sleeping, and safe surrender of abandoned infants. Intake of cases expanded from homicide cases to deaths caused by all mechanisms of preventable injury. With time, teams developed and utilized reports, public education, child grief support, and occasional review of nonfatal cases.

Major federal input began with the United States Advisory Board on Child Abuse and Neglect's 1995 report, *"A Nation's Shame, Fatal Child Abuse and Neglect in the United States"*.[5,6] The Board had published other significant reports, but this report received national media attention. No components of the reports were adopted by government leaders, however. This was the final report before the Board was discontinued for budgetary reasons.

National agencies and associations had little activity until this century when the American Academy of Pediatrics, the Centers for Disease Control and Prevention, the National Association for Medical Examiners, the Department of Defense, and the Health Resources Services Administration advocated for and helped create CFR and prevention programs with federal funding.

COMMON STRUCTURES AND PURPOSE

Effective CFR teams have fairly common components that have been, respectively, reproduced or avoided for various reasons.

Membership includes a spectrum of core professions with a mix of others, including occasional political appointments. The type of membership often differs depending on whether the team is local or statewide.

Inclusive intake begins with all potentially suspicious or preventable child deaths identified through various agency data sources such as medical examiner/coroner data and public health data (vital statistics, death and birth certificates). Some teams review all child deaths. Systematic review involves multiple agencies sharing information one case at time. Some reviews may be extended to piece the facts of the death together into a tangible story. Follow-up data and published reports support team focus and accountability. And finally, exceptions to these structures provide both additional useful structures and some hazards.

MEMBERSHIP

Members usually represent the front-line process from their respective agencies. The ideal review involves the individuals who managed the case being reviewed. The core professions that usually are included in all review teams are the coroner/medical examiner, law enforcement, prosecutors, child protection social workers, medical providers (typically from pediatrics), public health, nursing, and other representatives from human service agencies. Others disciplines are often added, including education, civil attorneys, mental health, child abuse prevention advocates, clergy, and data collection experts.

INTAKE

Case intake can include all cases identified as confirmed or suspicious for child abuse, all deaths identified as preventable, or all child deaths. Some review teams screen cases to create a manageable caseload for team review. Intake may be delayed months and even years or may be as rapid as on the day of the death. Small counties may review all child deaths in their respective area or may join with other counties to form regional review teams to maximize resources and increase the efficiency in reviewing cases.

REVIEW

Some teams review cases systematically and fill out data collection forms. A longer, more comprehensive review can focus more on the details of the death to gain a better understanding of the circumstances leading to a death. Specific meetings can be convened more acutely to review cases pending investigations or autopsy results. Subcommittees may address specific circumstances including suicides, homicides, motor vehicle crashes, or neonatal cases or to develop prevention programs in their communities.

FOLLOW-UP

Follow-up of case review, data collection, and analysis connects a team with case outcomes. Data collection and analysis can take considerable time (eg, delay for a pending criminal case outcome), but these data can be added later to database systems, and the review team can be updated when case resolution occurs. All agencies involved can be measured and evaluated. Providing a measure of case outcome defines an agency as a member of the peer group. Failure or refusal to provide data hinders the entire process. Data analysis provides a baseline and direction for prevention efforts, and team reports assist in educating the community. Teams can compare their work with that of other teams of similar size. Sample reports and data from local and state teams can be viewed in the virtual library.[7]

EXCEPTIONS AND PROBLEMS

Some state teams do not review actual cases. This structure can free time to support local teams, but it denies the state team the lessons derived from the case review process. Some teams limit their intake of cases to those with previous CPS records. This intake process can miss homicides committed by caregivers who had had no current or previous CPS investigation. Some child homicide and most domestic violence fatality review (DVFR) teams avoid potential legal complications by reviewing cases in which court action has been finalized. The consequences of delayed adult review and delayed child review merits further analysis.

GROWTH, NEW RESOURCES, AND NEW CHALLENGES

The number of child death review teams grew from one team in 1978 to an estimated 1000 review teams with thousands of members in multiple countries (including the United States, Canada, Australia, New Zealand, the Philippines, Japan, Lebanon, Scotland, England, and Wales) in 2009, and other nations are initiating efforts. Most of these countries are affluent and have strong child abuse prevention programs, but other models are developing; in the Philippines, for example, a hospital-based model is being developed. The United Kingdom by law directed all boroughs to have child death review by April 2008. Israel and Lebanon had beginning forums that were interrupted by military conflict but reportedly have renewed their efforts. The World Health Organization includes child death review in its literature, and the International Society for Prevention of Child Abuse and Neglect has included child death review at international conferences.

Multiagency teams provide a wide spectrum of potentially vigorous resources. Professionals who had avoided topics such as child deaths and other issues relating to young children are brought together by the CFR process to work with professionals who address issues relating to children on a daily basis. The topic of death and the professions that address death have been added to the maze of agencies addressing child abuse. Coroners and medical examiners are augmented by law enforcement, prosecutors, and others who address the crime of homicide. Data systems that address death are connected to data for child abuse and neglect. This growing mix of agencies and themes brings a mixture of potential conflict and assured competence. Through this crucible of viewpoints and skills, a more vigorous and effective process is created.

Additional forums for infant and child death reviews followed in the 1980s and 1990s including fetal infant mortality review (FIMR), DVFR, and the latest, elder abuse fatality review. FIMR is a public health program to improve perinatal services. Cases are reviewed by health professionals, and data are provided on service problems, including cultural bias and limited health access. The results are used to advocate for system improvement. A national FIMR network is supported by the American College of Obstetrics and Gynecology (www.acog.org).[8] DVFR has grown with support from criminal justice systems. Teams are supported by the National Domestic Violence Fatality Review Initiative, whose website can be viewed at http://www.ndvfri.org.[9] Many states have this type of review process, generally with limitations on case intake to avoid cases with active criminal court action. Some joint review has brought DVFR and CFR teams together when a family has both child and adult fatalities. The case intake for elder abuse fatality review is unique, with the potential to address family or residential care programs.[10]

Comparison of various child and other death review systems provides lessons about criteria for intake, team membership, data systems, criminal investigation, and primary prevention. The network of teams continues to be a major mutual resource. The first major text, *Child Fatality Review* was published in 2007.[11] In response to the increased knowledge necessary to be expert in child abuse, the American Board of Pediatrics has created a subspecialty board in Child Abuse Pediatrics to begin in 2009. A key component of this specialty is knowledge about and participation on child death review teams. Expertise in child abuse also has developed in the arenas of mental health and nursing, including specialists in forensic interviews, nurse practitioner specialists, and other investigators.

CHANGING CULTURAL ATTITUDES ABOUT DEATH CAUSED BY CHILD ABUSE

Success and failure can motivate community change, but the actual change may be delayed until larger social and cultural institutions are ready to accept a new process. New programs may interact to create a change in the larger culture.

The "engine" that drives child death review includes the pain and distress caused by the death of a child. The news of these deaths also affects the community. The ability to temper that pain can come from working with a group in which others share in the pain. This personal support can make the process safer for professionals. Expanded public involvement and education follow media stories of fatal abuse and public education by review teams. This process can be particularly useful in developing prevention programs to help educate and inspire the public to support programs for preventing injury and violence.

News stories about fatal child abuse became more prominent in the 1990s. These stories have increased in frequency and expand from stories of family violence to stories about failure of CPS agencies to keep children safe. The focus on television changed from the heroic defense attorney to the heroic prosecutor. Occasionally, now, a medical examiner or forensic expert is a major character. Child abuse is a frequent theme in these programs, occasionally extending to include fatal abuse. The many forms of media, including the Internet, television programs, and movies, have reported on or used child death in various ways. One could argue that such use of this topic is exploitive; on the other hand, this media use has raised the public awareness of child death and its many causes.

SUCCESS, FAILURE, AND TWENTY-FIRST CENTURY CHALLENGES

The Internet provides increased access to information and information retrieval. Data collection systems, including those for vital statistics and hospital discharge data, are accessible with authorization. One objection is that these tools used in the CFR process may jeopardize personal privacy. It can be argued effectively that protection of records may come at the expense of child safety and injury prevention. The balance between protecting children and protecting records continues to be debated, and both have merit.

Cases that are reviewed may cross county lines and regions, and review teams have learned how to follow data trails to retrieve information. Some DVFR and CFR teams have varied their types of review, forming joint review teams as needed. The difference in case intake timelines makes these reviews problematic, but both these issues must be addressed, and the review process will improve with time.

Tension often exists between human service and criminal justice systems. Agencies may choose to avoid conflict but may lose a potential resource that comes with collaboration and pursuing excellence in the CFR process with input from a peer group. Teams that face up to disagreements can be more vigorous and effective as professionals learn the potential value of others' expertise and knowledge.

The CFR movement also has influenced the development of multiple national data systems, including the Maternal Child Health National Center for Child Death Review[12] and a National Violent Death Data System (NVDRS) at the Centers for Disease Control and Prevention The ultimate goal of NVDRS is to provide communities with a clearer understanding of violent deaths so these deaths can be prevented. A wealth of information on this project can be found at the NVDRS website.[13]

National training in the investigation of sudden, unexpected infant death has increased the expertise of professionals who investigate infant death. Internet-based protocols and educational tools for coroners now are available. Increased interaction with people and programs outside the team, including news media, public education systems, and many local governmental agencies, has led to a national awareness of the CFR process. Some states have formed ombudsman offices that advocate for a balance of power among and an accountability of systems that are charged with the protection of children. Even more importantly, CFR has added to the knowledge base of professionals who help children who are survivors of family violence. Knowledge about child victims needs to be collected and shared, as well as what little is known about those rare young children who have committed homicides. Communication systems need to be developed that can share and link these uncommon cases to pool and increase knowledge about how to address similar cases. In addition, the need for grief support for child survivors identified through systematic review of cases is an important lesson learned from CFR. Multiple teams have begun to review nonfatal severe child injuries. Different jurisdictions and systems are connecting across nations.

There are still problems with agencies and individuals resisting the process of working together. Because of personal or system repercussions after problems are identified, agencies and individuals may find it easier to protect themselves rather than protect the children they serve. Cultural changes have occurred and expanded with peer support and the realization that quality improvement comes with acknowledgment of mistakes or failures. The failures to protect children from abusive death are real, but so are the many successes that have changed this culture of isolation and self protection. The collaborative nature of CFR embraces professionals who are willing to provide peer support and monitor peer accountability.

PEDIATRICIANS AND CHILD FATALITY REVIEW

Although state laws require autopsy in sudden, unexpected deaths or suspicious deaths of young children, many children die in circumstances in which no autopsy is done. In these cases (eg, in nearly all neonatal deaths), the pediatrician ascertains the cause of death and completes the death certificate. Whether the CFR team reviews potential child abuse cases or all causes of child death, the pediatrician usually is involved. Pediatricians' expertise in a variety of causes of death, and particularly the expertise of child abuse pediatricians in the range of child abuse, makes them key members of the fatality review team.

The American Academy of Pediatrics has made a number of recommendations regarding the investigation of child deaths and the role of the pediatrician:[14]

1. Advocating for proper death certification for children
2. Supporting state legislation requiring autopsies for unexpected or suspicious deaths
3. Supporting state legislation establishing CFR at the local and state levels and helping establish such teams
4. Serving on such committees and supporting other groups/agencies interested in such review
5. Becoming involved in the training of death scene investigators and serving as a consultant
6. Supporting state chapter and national initiatives aimed at reducing child deaths
7. Supporting calls for an increase in the supply of trained professionals; major enhancement of joint training by government agencies and professional organizations; encouraging states, military branches, and Indian Nations to implement joint criminal investigation teams; and encouraging the federal government to keep the documentation and prevention of child deaths as a priority.

SUMMARY

Groups of people gathering to study death is not a new phenomenon. Primitive people probably shared their fears when a member of the tribe died. Today, child death review has the unique feature of multiple agencies cooperating in one basic process. Children continue to die, and their deaths generate emotional pain that can increase multiagency cooperation. Child death review requires both the coordinated service and the accountability of a working peer group. Both the general pediatrician and the child abuse expert contribute to the CFR process and collaborate with these many child welfare professionals.

Teams have spread internationally with few resources, and much of that expansion has come from the efforts of individuals and small groups that persist with their action, inspired, in part, by the death of children as a personal issue and by the desire to prevent other deaths from happening. Tardieu's prescient work is evidence of the limits of unwanted knowledge. Changing attitudes currently allow topics to be addressed that previously were denied and professions to connect that previously were kept separate. In some ways this process may have recreated the personal ties that may have occurred more in primitive societies. This personal network coupled with new technologies fosters broad human connections and allows a growing mass of information about child death review to be shared both nationally and internationally.

REFERENCES

1. Tardieu A. Etude medico-legale sur les services et mauvais traitments exerces sur les enfants. Ann D Hyg Publ et Med-Leg 1860;13:361–98.
2. Kempe CH, Silverman FH, Steele BF, et al. The battered child syndrome. JAMA 1962;181:17–24.

3. Durfee M. Introduction In: Child fatality review: an interdisciplinary guide and photographic reference. St Louis: GW Medical; 2007. p. xv–xvi.
4. U.S. Department of Health and Human Services. Administration on children, youth and families. Child maltreatment 2006. Washington, DC: U.S. Department of Health and Human Services; 2008. Available at: http://www.acf.hhs.gov/programs/cb/stats_research/index.htm#can.
5. United States Advisory Board on Child Abuse and Neglect, U.S. Department of Health and Human Services, 1995. A nation's shame: fatal child abuse and neglect in the United States. Available at: http://www.ican-ncfr.org/documents/Nations-Shame.pdf.
6. Durfee D. Child death review teams: examples and overview. In: Child fatality review: an interdisciplinary guide and photographic reference. St Louis: GW Medical; 2007. p. 503–12.
7. The National Center of Child Fatality Review. Available at: http://www.ican-ncfr.org/resVirtualLibrary.asp.
8. American College of Obstetrics and Gynecology. Available at: http://www.acog.org/departments/dept_web.cfm?recno=10.
9. National Domestic Violence Fatality Review Initiative. Available at: http://www.ndvfri.org.
10. The National Center on Child Fatality Review. Elder abuse fatality review. Available at: http://www.ican-ncfr.org/hmElderAbuseFatality.asp.
11. Alexander R. Child fatality review: an interdisciplinary guide and photographic reference. St Louis: GW Medical; 2007.
12. Maternal Child Health National Center for Child Death Review. Available at: http://www.childdeathreview.org.
13. Department of Health and Human Services, Centers for Disease Control and Prevention. National violent death reporting system. Available at: http://www.cdc.gov/ncipc/profiles/nvdrs/default.htm.
14. American Academy of Pediatrics. Committee on Child Abuse and Neglect and Committee on Community Health Services. Investigation and review of unexpected infant and child deaths. Pediatrics 1999;104:1158–60.

Home Visiting for the Prevention of Child Maltreatment: Lessons Learned During the Past 20 Years

Nancy Donelan-McCall, PhD[a],*, John Eckenrode, PhD[b,c],
David L. Olds, PhD[a,d,e,f,g]

KEYWORDS

- Home visiting • Child maltreatment • Prevention
- Nurses • Policy • Early childhood

During the past 20 years, one of the most promising prevention strategies targeted at decreasing rates of child maltreatment has been to provide health services, parenting education, and social support to pregnant women and families with young children in their own homes. During the late 1970s and early 1980s several home visitation programs were developed and examined using both quasi-experimental and experimental designs. Preliminary findings were quite promising. As a result, home visitation programs were promoted as a means of improving the outcomes of pregnancy and reducing rates of infant mortality and morbidity (including reductions in child maltreatment). Subsequent reviews of the literature on home visiting programs have produced both sobering pictures of the prospects for home visiting programs in general[1–3] and

[a] Department of Pediatrics, University of Colorado Denver, 13121 E. 17th Avenue, Mail Stop 8410, Aurora, CO 80045, USA
[b] Department of Human Development, College of Human Ecology, G21 Martha Van Rensselaer Hall, Cornell University, Ithaca, NY 14853, USA
[c] Family Life Development Center, Cornell University, G21 Martha Van Rensselaer Hall, Ithaca, NY 14853, USA
[d] Department of Psychiatry, University of Colorado Denver, 13121 E. 17th Avenue, Mail Stop 8410, Aurora, CO 80045, USA
[e] Department of Nursing, University of Colorado Denver, 13121 E. 17th Avenue, Mail Stop 8410, Aurora, CO 80045, USA
[f] Department of Preventive Medicine, University of Colorado Denver, 13121 E. 17th Avenue, Mail Stop 8410, Aurora, CO 80045, USA
[g] Prevention Research Center for Family and Child Health, University of Colorado Denver, Aurora, CO, USA
* Corresponding author.
E-mail address: nancy.donelan-mccall@ucdenver.edu (N. Donelan-McCall).

Pediatr Clin N Am 56 (2009) 389–403
doi:10.1016/j.pcl.2009.01.002
0031-3955/09/$ – see front matter © 2009 Elsevier Inc. All rights reserved.

more optimistic evaluations of particular home visitation programs as means of preventing child abuse and neglect.[4,5]

This article examines how the field of home visitation for the prevention of child maltreatment has evolved during the past 29 years. It reviews the history and most recent findings from several home visitation programs focused on the prevention of child maltreatment. It gives particular attention to programs evaluated in randomized, controlled trials and highlights the Nurse-Family Partnership (NFP) program. It discusses how advocacy and public policy for the prevention of child maltreatment have shifted from a general call to promote universal home visitation to a more refined emphasis on promoting programs that are evidenced based, targeted to those most at risk for maltreatment, and with infrastructure in place to ensure implementation with fidelity to the model tested in trials. Finally, it discusses how primary care providers may advocate to ensure that their patients have access to evidence-based home visiting programs that meet their needs.

EVOLUTION OF HOME VISITING PROGRAMS

In the 1970s and 1980s, concerns regarding increasing rates of child maltreatment and growing numbers of children who were not "ready" to begin school spurred the development of several independent home visitation models for pregnant women and families with young children. These programs shared a common commitment to improve parents' early care of their children, but other features of the programs differed substantially. Home visiting programs differ in the backgrounds of the visitors, the segments of the parent population they target, the specific content and clinical methods of the programs, and the structure provided to the visitors in delivering the services. The following sections describe some of the better-established and well-researched programs developed during the 1970s and early 80s.

Hawaii Healthy Start Program

In 1975, the Hawaii Healthy Start Program (HSP) began as a single site on the Island of Oahu. The program targeted families with newborns thought to be at risk of child abuse and neglect. Trained paraprofessionals conducted home visits for the child's first 3 to 5 years, depending on family need.[6] HSP sought to address existing family crises, link families to needed services, promote child health and development through parent education, increase parents' skill in interacting with their children, model problem solving, and identify a medical home for each child.[6]

Although there was no evaluation of the program, six HSP home visitation programs were launched on other Hawaiian islands, and in 1984 the Hawaii state legislature authorized funding for additional program development and an evaluation of an HSP program on Oahu. This non-experimental evaluation found that graduates of the program had much lower rates of child maltreatment (< 3%) than did families with similar social characteristics not enrolled in the program. These findings led to a statewide expansion of the program.

Parents as Teachers

The Parents as Teachers (PAT) program began in 1981 in Missouri and grew out of the work of Burton White, who emphasized the importance of parenting during the first 3 years of life for later learning and success.[7] PAT is a universal parent-education program delivered by trained parent educators who begin working with parents either during pregnancy or soon after the child's birth and continue through the child's third birthday. The program consists of monthly home visits, parent group meetings, child development screenings, and referrals for services.

During the mid- to late-1980s, several quasi-experimental studies found that the children of parents who participated in PAT had fewer documented reports of child maltreatment compared with the Missouri state average. In addition, these studies found that children in PAT had better school readiness and that parents in PAT had better knowledge of child development and greater involvement in their children's education.[8,9]

Nurse-Family Partnership

The NFP program began in Elmira, New York in 1977 as an intervention tested in a randomized, controlled trial with a relatively large sample of low-income, primarily white, first-time mothers. The NFP has three goals: to improve the outcomes of pregnancy; to improve the child's subsequent health and development (in part by preventing child abuse and neglect); and to improve families' economic self-sufficiency. The NFP is grounded in epidemiology and theories of human ecology,[10] self-efficacy,[11] and human attachment.[12]

The NFP enrolled pregnant, low-income women having first births, a population with a large proportion of unmarried and adolescent mothers. These mothers are at higher risk for poor birth outcomes, child abuse and neglect, and diminished parental economic self-sufficiency.[13] Women bearing first children are particularly receptive to efforts to guide them to achieve better lives for their children and themselves. To the extent that they improve their prenatal health, care of their firstborns, and life-course, they are likely to apply those skills to subsequent children.[14] On average, mothers were scheduled to be seen every 2 weeks, with the frequency of home visits varying based on the stage of pregnancy and parents' needs.

Nurses, rather than paraprofessionals or social workers, were selected as home visitors because of their formal training in health care and their corresponding ability to address mothers' and family members' concerns about the complications of pregnancy, labor, and delivery, and the physical health of the infant. Their expertise was thought to increase nurses' credibility with family members.

The NFP conceptual model illustrates how the program aims to prevent child maltreatment through multiple pathways within the family system (**Fig. 1**). For example, to the extent that nurse visitations reduce women's use of tobacco and alcohol during pregnancy, they reduce the likelihood that children will be exposed to substances that can create perturbations in fetal brain development that, in turn, can make babies more irritable and difficult to parent.[15,16] The promotion of parents' competence in providing care that is sensitive and responsive fosters children's development. Parents who accurately read their babies' cues, empathize with their infants, and respond sensitively to their babies' signals are less likely to abuse or neglect their children and are more likely to read their children's developmental competencies accurately, leading to fewer unintentional injuries.[17] The nurses also worked closely with mothers around issues of fertility. Closely spaced subsequent births undermine unmarried women's educational achievement and workforce participation[18] and increase the risk for children's injuries,[19] probably because of compromised parental supervision.

Elmira results

The Elmira NFP trial was the first study to use a randomized, controlled design to examine the effects of home visitation on at-risk families. The 400 women enrolled in the trial were randomly assigned to receive either home visitation or comparison

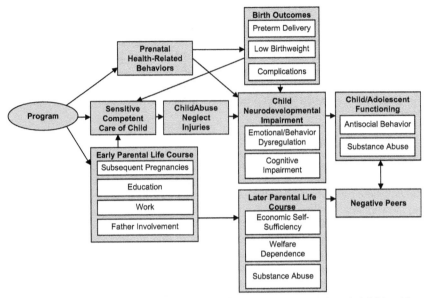

Fig. 1. General conceptual model of program influences on maternal and child health and development. (*From* Olds DL. Prenatal and infancy home visiting by nurses: from randomized trials to community replication. Prevention Science 2002;3(3);155; with permission from Springer Science and Business Media.)

services (health and developmental screenings with and without free transportation to prenatal and well-child visits). Initial findings from the Elmira trial were quite promising.

During the first 2 years of the child's life, nurse-visited children born to low-income, unmarried teenaged mothers had 80% fewer verified cases of child abuse and neglect than did their counterparts in the control group (ie, one case [4%] in the low-income nurse-visited unmarried teenaged mothers, versus 8 cases [19%] in the control group, $P = .07$). **Fig. 2** shows that the treatment–control differences on verified reports of child maltreatment were greater among families where there was more concentrated social disadvantage. During the second year of life, nurse-visited children were seen in the emergency department 32% fewer times. This difference was explained in part by a 56% reduction in emergency department visits for injuries and ingestions. Although the effect of the program on substantiated rates of child abuse and neglect was only a trend, the program effect was corroborated by observations of mothers' treatment of their children in their homes and injuries detected in the children's medical records.[20]

During the 2-year period after the program ended, the beneficial impact of the NFP endured for many outcomes. Children of nurse-visited women were less likely than children in the comparison group to receive emergency room treatment and to visit a physician for injuries and ingestions.[21] The effect of the program on state-verified cases of child abuse and neglect, on the other hand, was not statistically significant during that 2-year period,[21] probably because of increased detection of child abuse and neglect in nurse-visited families and nurses' linkage of families with needed services (including child protective services) at the end of the program.

Maltreated children and their families who were nurse visited differed substantially from maltreated children and their families in the comparison group. For example, in contrast to maltreated children in the comparison group, nurse-visited maltreated children paid 38% fewer visits to the emergency department and 87% fewer visits to

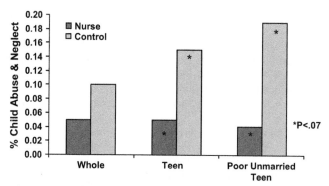

Fig. 2. Indicated cases of child abuse and neglect: 0 to 2 years, Elmira. Rates of verified cases of child abuse and neglect by treatment condition and socio-demographic characteristics of sample. (*From* Olds DL. Preventing child maltreatment and crime with prenatal and infancy support of parents: the Nurse-Family Partnership. Journal of Scandinavian Studies in Criminology and Crime Prevention 2008;9(1);9; with permission from the Taylor & Francis Group.)

a physician for injuries or ingestions from the twenty-fifth through the fiftieth month of life period.[22]

The Elmira trial found that the NFP affects a range of risk factors for child maltreatment and children's general health and well being. During pregnancy, nurse-visited women had greater reductions in smoking,[23] experienced greater informal social support, and made better use of formal community services.[23] At birth, nurse-visited women identified as smokers had 75% fewer preterm deliveries, and nurse-visited very young adolescents had higher birth weight babies than their control group counterparts.[23]

During the first 4 years of the child's life, parenting improved among nurse-visited poor, unmarried teens, in contrast to their counterparts in the control group. The nurse-visited mothers exhibited less punishment and restriction of their infants, provided more appropriate play materials, and provided safer, more developmentally conducive home environments.[21] Child development outcomes were improved for the children of nurse-visited women as opposed to comparison families. Children were less irritable and fussy during infancy,[24] and children of mothers who smoked during pregnancy were less likely to experience declines in intellectual functioning.[25]

Maternal life course improved for nurse-visited versus comparison families. Nurse-visited families had fewer subsequent pregnancies, longer intervals between births of first and second children, and greater participation in the work force.[26]

CALL FOR EXPANSION OF HOME VISITATION PROGRAMS

By the mid-1980s, small-scale quasi-experimental studies and a single randomized, controlled trial (the Elmira trial of the NFP) formed the evidentiary support for home visitation programs. Concerns about high rates of child maltreatment and infant mortality prompted the National Commission to Prevent Infant Mortality[27] to advocate in 1989 for the expansion of home visiting programs as a means of preventing infant mortality and for the US Advisory Board on Child Abuse and Neglect to recommend in 1991that a system of universal home visiting be established to prevent child maltreatment.[28] In 1998, the Council on Child and Adolescent Health of the American

Academy of Pediatrics[29] recommended that primary care be augmented with home visiting services for vulnerable children and families.

In response to the Advisory Board's recommendation, the National Committee to Prevent Child Abuse (known now as Prevent Child Abuse America) created Healthy Families America (HFA), a national initiative designed to disseminate the Hawaii HSP model throughout the United States. The program grew quickly, and in 2008 HFA programs were located in 440 locations throughout the United States and Canada.

Although largely based on the Hawaii HSP, the HFA model does not follow a specific set of guidelines or visitation protocols. Instead, the HFA model is defined by "its commitment to a set of principles rather than to a single, monolithic approach."[30] There are commonalities among most HFA programs: programs typically are delivered by paraprofessional home visitors; families deemed at risk for child abuse and neglect are enrolled during pregnancy or postpartum; primary prevention services are provided as well as services to families who have a previous history of child maltreatment; visits are conducted in families' homes until children are 3 to 5 years old, according to a visitation schedule that diminishes in frequency as families improve in their functioning; and the visitors focus on helping parents become more competent caregivers.

The PAT program also expanded rapidly during this period. The initial pilot work prompted the state of Missouri to implement the PAT program in all Missouri school districts. In 1990, the California state legislature created a grant program to implement PAT in selected communities, with the goal of targeting the program to parents and families who had limited English proficiency and to teen-aged parents.[31] Since 1985, PAT has expanded to all 50 states and to other countries.

During this same period, leadership of the NFP received repeated requests to offer this program for public investment but declined until evidence was available from additional randomized, controlled trials that replicated the promising results from the Elmira trial with diverse populations living in a variety of contexts.

RECENT RESEARCH ON HOME VISITING PROGRAMS

Following dissemination efforts of HFA and PAT, concerns regarding the lack of evidence to support these programs led to the conduct of several randomized, controlled trials of each model in a variety of communities. In addition, in recent years other home visiting models targeted at reducing child maltreatment were developed and evaluated through randomized, controlled trials. During the past 2 decades, Olds and his colleagues have conducted two additional trials of the NFP program and continued to follow the Elmira families. The following sections present the results of more recent research trials of home visitation programs.

Healthy Families America

Since the widespread dissemination effort of the Hawaiian HSP model (through HFA), a series of randomized, controlled trials has been conducted on the HSP program and its HFA spin-offs. Because the HFA model relies on a set of principles rather than on a structured model, each HFA program is a separate initiative or program model. This variability complicates the interpretation of program impacts across sites and generalizations to different settings and populations.

The authors summarize findings from four randomized, controlled trials of HFA programs implemented in New York, Alaska, San Diego, and Hawaii. Two of the trials showed small effects for some self-reported parenting behaviors that are associated with child abuse and neglect (reports of abusive behaviors).[32,33] Across all four trials, no effects have been found on measures of childhood injuries or other objectively measured outcomes consistent with the prevention of maltreatment. Program effects on observed features of the environment, child development, and parent reporting of child behavior at age 2 years were found in one trial,[34] but a corresponding effect on child development in a different trial did not endure.[35] In the New York evaluation, program effects on self-reports of serious abuse and neglect were greater for a prevention group (families registered during pregnancy with mothers younger than 19 years of age having a first child) and for mothers who were more psychologically vulnerable.[33]

Very few effects were found across all trials with regard to mother's life course, stress, or psychological well being. Overall, findings from trials of the HFA model have been disappointing.[4,36,37] HFA also seems not to be cost effective. The Washington State Institute for Public Policy[38] has estimated that an investment in HFA produces a loss of $1830 for each family. Poor implementation has been offered as an explanation for the limited outcomes found in two of these trials (in Alaska and Hawaii).[6] At least one of the trials (in San Diego) was well implemented, but the findings still were disappointing. Bugental and her colleagues[39] have implemented an experimental approach to enhancing HFA that shows promise in improving parenting behaviors based on self-report.

Parents as Teachers

Four separate randomized, controlled trials have been conducted of the PAT program since the program began dissemination efforts: one designed to examine program impacts in families who had limited English proficiency;[31] one to examine PAT impacts on teen-aged parents;[31] a trial of PAT in three communities;[31] and a fourth trial that examined whether the Born to Learn (BTL) curriculum would enhance PAT and produce an impact on children's development (D. Drotar, unpublished data, 2006).

Findings from the first two randomized, controlled trials did not produce consistently promising results. In one trial, as reflected in official records, parents in the PAT program had fewer instances of child maltreatment.[31] The low rates of opened cases (2.4% in the control group), low rates of research retention, and statistical concerns decrease confidence in this finding. There were no clinically meaningful impacts of PAT on measures of child development or observations of the home environment pertinent to child maltreatment outcomes. Although parents reported improved child development and parenting in some trials, no program impacts were found on objective measures of children's cognitive functioning or behavior.

The multisite trial of PAT found few statistically significant effects on parenting or child outcomes. PAT mothers reported being "very happy" while caring for their child at the 2-year assessment. There were no overall differences in mothers' knowledge of child development or parents' reports of their observations of their children. PAT mothers had higher scores on a measure of language- and literacy-promoting behaviors, but there were no overall program effects on any of the child outcomes.[40] Finally, a fourth randomized, controlled trial examining the impacts of PAT with BTL found improvements in children's mastery motivation and teachers' rating of child assertion (D. Drotar, unpublished data, 2006), but there were no overall program effects on children's cognitive development, attachment security, or conceptual skills or on parents' knowledge of child development or sense of competence.

Researchers have been evaluating ways to improve the PAT model through curriculum development and testing, a commendable approach. The Washington State

Institute for Public Policy has determined that Parents as Teachers produces a savings of $1509 per family.[38]

Early Intervention Program

Deborah Koniak-Griffin and colleagues[41–44] designed and evaluated a program of nurse home visiting known as the Early Intervention Program (EIP). The program targets first-time adolescent mothers and focuses on improving pregnancy outcomes and child health and development by improving parents' care of their children and maternal life-course. Nurses began visiting in mid-pregnancy (20 weeks) and continued through the infants' first 12 months of life. This program is similar in conceptual background and delivery to the NFP, but there are several distinct differences. In the EIP, nurses had other caseload responsibilities in addition to the EIP, nurses met with mothers in groups during pregnancy, the program was shorter in duration (12 versus 24 months postpartum), and the nurses visited less frequently.

Findings from two published reports of this trial are promising for preventing child maltreatment. At 6 weeks postpartum, compared with infants assigned to a traditional public health nursing group (two visits during pregnancy and one postnatal visit), EIP infants had fewer days in the hospital and fewer total episodes of hospitalizations involving injuries; program effects continued up to 24 months.[42–44] At 1 year, the EIP infants demonstrated significantly higher rates of immunizations, but there were no other significant program effects on mother–child interaction, subsequent pregnancies, maternal depression, or substance use.[44]

Given the short duration (and corresponding reduced cost) of this program, it would be useful to see whether it produces effects on other clinically important aspects of maternal and child functioning (eg, mental health, maternal employment, father involvement, and qualities of parent–child interaction) and whether the program is cost effective in the long term.[45]

Nurse Home Visitation for Prevention of Recidivism of Child Maltreatment

MacMillan and her colleagues[46] investigated whether a nurse home visitation program targeted at families in which the target child had been exposed to physical abuse or neglect would be effective in preventing the recurrence of child maltreatment. Families with a child younger than 13 years of age who had a reported episode of physical abuse or neglect within the past 3 months and still residing with the family were assigned randomly to either the intervention program or a control group. Intervention families received nurse home visitation every week for 6 months, then every 2 weeks for 6 months, then monthly for 12 months. Nurses focused on decreasing stressors and increasing support by tailoring the home visits to the needs of the family, addressing parent education about child development, and providing links to community health and social service resources. Families in the standard-care control group were given routine follow-up by child protection service caseworkers, parent education, and referrals to community-based parenting education.

Three years after enrollment (1 year after intervention), there were no differences between the treatment and the control groups in child protection agency reports of physical abuse or neglect. The intervention group, however, had higher rates of physical abuse or neglect documented in hospital records.[46] Although nurse home visitation models have been effective in preventing the initiation of child maltreatment,[47] this trial emphasizes just how hard it is to transform parenting once dysfunctional patterns have been set in motion.[46] Some parent-training approaches, such as Project Safecare, show promise in reducing maltreatment recidivism, but Project Safecare has not been tested in a randomized, controlled trial; evidence from randomized, controlled trials is needed before this program warrants public investment.[48]

Nurse-Family Partnership

Following the initial findings from the Elmira NFP trial, the lead investigators of the NFP continued to develop and test the NFP in randomized trials to ensure that the program had enduring effects on clinically important outcomes across diverse populations and contexts before offering the program for public investment. Toward this goal they conducted additional trials in Memphis, Tennessee and Denver, Colorado. In addition, they continued to follow the original Elmira sample into early adulthood.

Although the nature of the home visitation services was essentially the same in each of the trials, as described earlier, the samples and comparison services were different. The Memphis sample was primarily black. The Denver trial consisted of a large sample of Hispanics and included, in addition to nurses, an experimental group that examined the impact of the program when delivered by paraprofessionals. In all the trials, the control group received services above and beyond those currently available, such as transportation for routine prenatal care and infant developmental screening and referral for further evaluation and treatment.

Memphis results

The rate of substantiated child abuse and neglect in the population of 2-year-old, low-income children in Memphis was too low (3%–4%) to serve as a valid indicator of child maltreatment in this study. The investigators hypothesized instead that program effects would emerge for childhood injuries, similar to the observations in Elmira. Moreover, they hypothesized that program effects on childhood injuries would be more prominent among children born to mothers who were psychologically vulnerable. During their first 2 years of life, compared with children in the comparison group, nurse-visited children had 23% fewer health care encounters for injuries and ingestions and were hospitalized for 79% fewer days with injuries and/or ingestions, effects that, as predicted, were more pronounced for children born to mothers whose psychological resources placed them in the lower half of the sample.[49]

Even though infant and childhood mortality are uncommon events, by age 9 years, children in the control group were 4.5 times more likely to have died than their counterparts in the nurse-visited group ($P < .08$). There were 10 deaths in the control group; one was not preventable (caused by multiple congenital anomalies), three were caused by preterm delivery; three were caused by sudden infant death syndrome; and three were caused by injury, including two by firearm. The one death in the nurse-visited group was caused by a chromosomal anomaly.[50] Along with findings from the Elmira trial, these results reinforce the interpretation that the program reduced the rates of grossly deficient care of children.

Findings from the Memphis trial support earlier findings from the Elmira trial, in that the program affected important risks for child maltreatment, including deficient caregiving and maternal life-course.[49]

Denver results

In the Denver trial, the investigators could not access women's or children's medical records to assess their injury encounters (as they had in Elmira and Memphis), because the health care delivery system was too complex to abstract all of their health care encounters reliably. Moreover, as in Memphis, the rate of state-verified reports of child abuse and neglect was too low in this population (3%–4% for low-income children between birth and 2 years of age) to use child protective service records to assess the impact of the program on child maltreatment. Therefore, this team devoted more resources to measuring the children's early emotional development.

The nurse visitations produced effects consistent with those achieved in earlier trials of the program. During the first 24 months of the child's life, nurse-visited mother-infant dyads interacted more responsively than did control pairs, and nurse-visited children had better language functioning and superior mental development at 2 and 4 years than control pairs, an effect concentrated in the group defined by mothers who were more psychologically vulnerable.[51,52] Nurse-visited women, compared with controls, were less likely to have had a subsequent pregnancy and birth, had longer intervals until the next conception,[51,52] and, at child age 4 years, experienced less domestic violence than women in the comparison group.[52]

While the program was in operation, for most outcomes on which there was an effect, paraprofessionals produced effects that were approximately half the size of those produced by nurses. Paraprofessional-visited mothers began to experience benefits from the program 2 years after the program ended at child age 2 years, but on most outcomes their children were not statistically distinguishable from their control-group counterparts.

Elmira 15-year follow-up results

Results from a 15-year follow-up of the Elmira sample[53] indicate that the program effects on state-verified reports of child abuse and neglect grew between the children's fourth and fifteenth birthdays. Overall, during the 15-year period after delivery of their first child, in contrast to women in the control group, those visited by nurses during pregnancy and infancy were identified as perpetrators of child abuse and neglect in an average of 0.29 (versus 0.54) verified reports per program participant, an effect that was greater for women who were poor and unmarried at registration.[53] The impact of the program on child abuse and neglect through child age 15 years was attenuated in the context of moderate to high levels of intimate partner violence.[54] Furthermore, for the 80% of mothers in the study who experienced low to moderate levels of domestic violence, the treatment effect on maltreatment reports at 15 years was mediated by fewer numbers of subsequent children and by fewer months on public assistance.[55]

Summarizing findings across the three trials of the NFP, the Washington Institute for Public Policy estimated that the NFP program, when implemented with nurse home visitors, saves $18,054 per family.[38]

REPLICATION AND SCALE-UP OF THE NURSE-FAMILY PARTNERSHIP

In 1996, the Department of Justice invited representatives of the NFP to replicate the program outside of research contexts. With the results of the Memphis trial showing essential replication of many of the major findings from the Elmira trial, this team accepted the invitation but built into the replication process a structure to help ensure that the program would be conducted with fidelity to the model tested in the trials. Even when communities choose to develop programs based on models with good scientific evidence, these programs run the risk of being watered down in the process of being scaled up.[56] The NFP National Service Office, a nonprofit organization, was created to help new communities replicate the NFP with fidelity to the model tested in the scientifically controlled studies.

Each site choosing to implement the NFP needs certain capacities to operate and sustain the program with high quality. These capacities include having an organization and community that are fully knowledgeable and supportive of the program, a staff that is well trained and well supported in the conduct of the program model, and real-time information on the program's achievement of implementation and maternal and child health benchmarks. These accountability data guide efforts to maintain and to improve continuously the quality of the program.

Today the program is operating in 350 counties nationally. State and local governments are securing financial support for the NFP (about $9500 per family for 2.5 years of services, in 2006 dollars) from existing sources of funds, such as Temporary Assistance to Needy Families, Medicaid, the Maternal and Child Health Block-Grant, and child-abuse and crime-prevention dollars. At present, research is being conducted to strengthen the NFP program in addressing issues such as intimate partner violence and maternal mental illness.

PUBLIC POLICY AND ADVOCACY IMPLICATIONS

Even though many questions need to be resolved, research during the past 20 years is beginning to provide a sufficiently coherent picture so that some policy and practice recommendations can be made with increasing confidence.

First, public investment in home visiting programs targeted at reducing child maltreatment should be allocated to evidence-based programs. Policy and practice recommendations for parenting interventions will be improved if they advocate programs found to produce enduring, replicated impacts of public health importance in randomized, controlled trials; if they advocate programs tested with different populations living in different contexts; if such programs have well-articulated implementation guidelines; and if such programs have established procedures to ensure reliable replication of program elements.

A recent funding announcement[57] from the Administration for Children and Youth (ACF) highlights growing policy commitment to allocating dollars to evidenced-based home visitation programs. This announcement provides funding to communities to develop the infrastructure for widespread adoption, implementation, and sustainability of evidenced-based home vitation programs targeted at the prevention of child maltreatment. This grant program provides specific guidelines for what constitutes an evidence-based program and outlines a policy that increases the probability that scarce public dollars will be allocated to programs that have a strong likelihood of preventing maltreatment.

One of the clearest messages from the NFP program of research, supported by findings from HFA and EIP, is that the functional and economic benefits of home visitation programs are greatest for families at greater risk. In Elmira, it was evident that most married women and those from higher socioeconomic households managed the care of their children without serious problems and were able to avoid lives of welfare dependence, substance abuse, and crime without the assistance of the nurse home-visitors. On the other hand, low-income, unmarried women and their children in the control group were at much greater risk for these problems, and the program was able to avert many of these untoward outcomes for this at-risk population. This pattern of results challenges the position that these intensive programs should be made available on a universal basis. Doing so is likely to be wasteful from an economic standpoint and may lead to a dilution of services for those families who need them most because of insufficient resources to serve everyone well.

Procedures need to be developed to ensure that the essential elements of evidence-based parenting programs can be implemented reliably in a variety of practice settings so that they will produce their intended effects. The recent ACF program announcement endorses this kind of standard. Furthermore, program evaluation needs to be on-going in community practice to ensure that programs continue to produce effects on targeted outcomes so that children, families, and communities receive the benefits they were promised.

ADVOCACY FOR THE PRIMARY CARE PROVIDER

The NFP has the strongest evidence that it can prevent child maltreatment of any home visiting program examined to date. In fact, two recent reviews of early childhood and early education interventions placed the NFP in the top tier of evidence-based interventions.[58,59] What can primary care providers do to support such a program? The authors believe that the evidence warrants reconsideration of the American Academy of Pediatrics, Council on Child and Adolescent Health recommendation on home visitation programs.[29] Given advances in the understanding of what interventions work for preventing child maltreatment and other adverse outcomes for vulnerable children and families, the authors recommend that a revised statement include language consistent with the ACF recommendations.

Primary care providers should be aware of and promote the establishment of home visitation programs in their community that meet these high evidentiary standards. In addition, they should establish on-going relationships with such programs. Effective programs can reduce risks and adverse outcomes for fetal, infant, and child health and development. Although the NFP is the one home visiting program that has met the highest scientific standards and has the resources to ensure effective community replication, the authors believe that additional research should be conducted to develop and test other home visiting programs to help vulnerable parents care competently for their children in their homes. Society has a responsibility to vulnerable children and families to ensure that scarce public dollars are directed toward programs that are evidence-based, applied to the studied population, and implemented with fidelity.

REFERENCES

1. Olds DL, Kitzman H. Review of research on home visiting for pregnant women and parents of young children. Future Child 1993;3(3):53–92.
2. Gomby DS, Culross PL, Behrman RE. Home visiting: recent program evaluations—analysis and recommendations. Future Child 1999;9(1):4–26, 195–223.
3. Sweet MA, Appelbaum MI. Is home visiting an effective strategy? A meta-analytic review of home visiting programs for families with young children. Child Dev 2004; 75:1435–56.
4. Krugman SD, Lane WG, Walsh CM. Update on child abuse prevention. Curr Opin Pediatr 2007;19(6):711–8.
5. Hahn RA, Bilukha OO, Crosby A, et al. First reports evaluating the effectiveness of strategies for preventing violence: firearms laws. Findings from the Task Force on Community Preventive Services. MMWR Recomm Rep 2003;52(RR-14):11–20.
6. Duggan AK, McFarlane EC, Windham AM, et al. Evaluation of Hawaii's Healthy Start Program. Future Child 1999;9(1):66–90 [discussion: 177–8].
7. White B. The first three years of life. Indianapolis (IN): Prentice Hall Profession Technical Reference; 1985.
8. Winter M, McDonald D. Parents as teachers: investing in good beginnings for children. In: Albee G, Gullotta T, editors. Primary prevention works. Thousand Oaks (CA): Sage Publications; 1997. p. 119–45.
9. Pfannenstiel J, Seltzer D. Evaluation report: new parents as teachers project. Overland Park (KS): Research & Training Associates; 1985.

10. Bronfenbrenner U. The ecology of human development: experiments by nature and design. Cambridge (MA): Harvard University Press; 1979.

11. Bandura A. Self-efficacy: toward a unifying theory of behavioral change. Psychol Rev 1977;84(2):191–215.

12. Bowlby J. Attachment and loss, vol. 1. Attachment. New York: Basic Books; 1969.

13. Elster AB, McAnarney ER. Medical and psychosocial risks of pregnancy and childbearing during adolescence. Pediatr Ann 1980;9(3):89–94.

14. Olds DL. Prenatal and infancy home visiting by nurses: from randomized trials to community replication. Prevention Science 2002;2(3):153–72.

15. Shenassa ED, Brown MJ. Maternal smoking and infantile gastrointestinal dysregulation: the case of colic. Pediatrics 2004;114(4):e497–505.

16. Day NL, Richardson GA, Goldschmidt L, et al. Effects of prenatal tobacco exposure on preschoolers' behavior. J Dev Behav Pediatr 2000;21(3):180–8.

17. Peterson L, Gable S. Holistic injury prevention. In: Lutzker JR, editor. Handbook of child abuse research and treatment. New York: Plenum Press; 1998. p. 291–318.

18. Furstenberg FF, Brooks-Gunn J, Morgan SP. Adolescent mothers in later life. Cambridge (MA): Cambridge University Press; 1987.

19. Nathens AB, Neff MJ, Goss CH, et al. Effect of an older sibling and birth interval on the risk of childhood injury. Inj Prev 2000;6(3):219–22.

20. Olds DL. Preventing child maltreatment and crime with prenatal and infancy support of parents: the Nurse-Family Partnership. J Scand Stud Criminol Crime Prev 2008;9(1):2–24.

21. Olds DL, Henderson CR Jr, Kitzman H. Does prenatal and infancy nurse home visitation have enduring effects on qualities of parental caregiving and child health at 25 to 50 months of life? Pediatrics 1994;93(1):89–98.

22. Olds D, Henderson CR Jr, Kitzman H, et al. Effects of prenatal and infancy nurse home visitation on surveillance of child maltreatment. Pediatrics 1995;95(3):365–72.

23. Olds DL, Henderson CR Jr, Tatelbaum R, et al. Improving the delivery of prenatal care and outcomes of pregnancy: a randomized trial of nurse home visitation. Pediatrics 1986;77(1):16–28 [Erratum Appears in Pediatrics 1986 Jul;78(1):138].

24. Olds DL, Henderson CR Jr, Chamberlin R, et al. Preventing child abuse and neglect: a randomized trial of nurse home visitation. Pediatrics 1986;78(1):65–78.

25. Olds DL, Henderson CR Jr, Tatelbaum R. Prevention of intellectual impairment in children of women who smoke cigarettes during pregnancy. Pediatrics 1994;93(2):228–33 [Erratum appears in Pediatrics 1994;93(6 Pt 1):973].

26. Olds DL, Henderson CR Jr, Tatelbaum R, et al. Improving the life-course development of socially disadvantaged mothers: a randomized trial of nurse home visitation. Am J Public Health 1988;78(11):1436–45.

27. National Commission to Prevent Infant Mortality. Home visiting: opening doors for America's pregnant women and children. Washington, DC: National Commission to Prevent Infant Mortality; 1989.

28. US Advisory Board on Child Abuse and Neglect. Creating caring communities: blueprint for an effective federal policy on child abuse and neglect. Washington, DC: US Government Printing Office; 1991.

29. American Academy of Pediatrics: Council on Child and Adolescent Health. The role of home-visitation programs in improving health outcomes for children and families. Pediatrics 1998;101(3 Pt 1):486–9.

30. Daro DA, Harding KA. Healthy Families America: using research to enhance practice. Future Child 1999;9(1):152–78.

31. Wagner MM, Clayton SL. The Parents as Teachers program: results from two demonstrations. Future Child 1999;9(1):91–115, 179–89.

32. Mitchell-Herzfeld S, Izzo C, Greene R, et al. Evaluation of Healthy Families New York (HFNY): first year program impacts. New York: Office of Children and Family Bureau of Evaluation and Research; 2005.

33. DuMont K, Mitchell-Herzfeld S, Greene R, et al. Healthy Families New York (HFNY) randomized trial: impacts on parenting after the first two years. New York: New York State Office of Children & Family Services; 2006.

34. Duggan A, Rodriguez K, Burrell L, et al. Evaluation of the Healthy Families Alaska Program. Available at: http://www.hss.state.ak.us/ocs/Publications/JohnsHopkins_HealthyFamilies.pdf. Accessed March 31, 2008.

35. Landsverk J, Carrilio T, Connelly CD, et al. Healthy Families San Diego Clinical Trial technical report. San Diego (CA): Child and Adolescent Services Research Center, San Diego Children's Hospital and Health Center; 2002.

36. Chaffin M. Is it time to rethink Healthy Start/Healthy Families? Child Abuse Negl 2004;28(6):589–95.

37. Olds DL, Sadler L, Kitzman H. Programs for parents of infants and toddlers: recent evidence from randomized trials. J Child Psychol Psychiatry 2007; 48(3/4):355–91.

38. Lee S, Aos S, Miller M. Evidence-based programs to prevent children from entering and remaining in the child welfare system: benefits and costs for Washington. Document No. 08-07-3901. Olympia (WA): Washington State Institute for Public Policy; 2008.

39. Bugental DB, Ellerson PC, Lin EK, et al. A cognitive approach to child abuse prevention. J Fam Psychol 2002;16:243–58.

40. Wagner M, Iida E, Spiker D. The multisite evaluation of the Parents as Teachers home visiting program: three year findings from one community. Menlo Park (CA): SRI International; 2001.

41. Koniak-Griffin D, Anderson NL, Brecht ML, et al. Public health nursing care for adolescent mothers: impact on infant health and selected maternal outcomes at 1 year postbirth. J Adolesc Health 2002;30(1):44–54.

42. Koniak-Griffin D, Mathenge C, Anderson NL, et al. An early intervention program for adolescent mothers: a nursing demonstration project. J Obstet Gynecol Neonatal Nurs 1999;28(1):51–9.

43. Koniak-Griffin D, Anderson NL, Verzemnieks I, et al. A public health nursing early intervention program for adolescent mothers: outcomes from pregnancy through 6 weeks postpartum. Nurse Res 2000;49(3):130–8.

44. Koniak-Griffin D, Verzemnieks IL, Anderson NL, et al. Nurse visitation for adolescent mothers: two-year infant health and maternal outcomes. Nurse Res 2003; 52(2):127–36.

45. Karoly LA, Kilburn MR, Cannon JS. Early childhood interventions: proven results, future promise. Santa Monica (CA): RAND; 2005.

46. MacMillan HL, Thomas BH, Jamieson E, et al. Effectiveness of home visitation by public-health nurses in prevention of the recurrence of child physical abuse and neglect: a randomised controlled trial. Lancet 2005;365(9473): 1786–93.

47. Olds DL. The Nurse-Family Partnership: an evidence-based preventive intervention. Infant Ment Health J 2006;27(1):5–25.

48. Gershater-Molko RM, Lutzker JR, Wesch D. Using recidivism data to evaluate Project Safecare: teaching bonding, safety, and health care skills to parents. Child Maltreat 2002;7(3):277–85.

49. Kitzman H, Olds DL, Henderson CR Jr, et al. Effect of prenatal and infancy home visitation by nurses on pregnancy outcomes, childhood injuries, and repeated childbearing. A randomized controlled trial. JAMA 1997;278(8): 644–52.

50. Olds DL, Kitzman H, Hanks C, et al. Effects of nurse home visiting on maternal and child functioning: age-9 follow-up of a randomized trial. Pediatrics 2007; 120(4):e832–45.

51. Olds DL, Robinson J, O'Brien R, et al. Home visiting by paraprofessionals and by nurses: a randomized, controlled trial. Pediatrics 2002;110(3):486–96.

52. Olds DL, Robinson J, Pettitt L, et al. Effects of home visits by paraprofessionals and by nurses: age-four follow-up of a randomized trial. Pediatrics 2004;114: 1560–8.

53. Olds DL, Eckenrode J, Henderson CR Jr, et al. Long-term effects of home visitation on maternal life course and child abuse and neglect. Fifteen-year follow-up of a randomized trial. JAMA 1997;278(8):637–43.

54. Eckenrode J, Ganzel B, Henderson CR Jr, et al. Preventing child abuse and neglect with a program of nurse home visitation: the limiting effects of domestic violence. JAMA 2000;284(11):1385–91.

55. Eckenrode J. Nurse home visitation as a prevention strategy. XIth ISPCAN European Conference on Child Abuse and Neglect. Lisbon, Portugal, November 8–21, 2007.

56. Olds DL, Hill PL, O'Brien R, et al. Taking preventive intervention to scale: the Nurse-Family Partnership. Cogn Behav Pract 2003;10(4):278–90.

57. Department of Health & Human Services Administration for Children and Families. Supporting evidence-based home visitation programs to prevent child maltreatment. Funding opportunity number HHS-2008-ACF-ACYF-CA-0130.

58. Coalition for Evidence-Based Policy. Initial results: congressionally-reviewed initiative to identify social programs backed by top tier evidence. On-line report. Available at: http://www.excelgov.org. Accessed December 5, 2008.

59. MacMillan HL, Wathen NC, Barlow J, et al. Interventions to prevent child maltreatment and associated impairment. Lancet 2008 Dec 3. Journal on-line. Available at: http://www.thelancet.com. Accessed December 5, 2008.

Achieving Better Health Care Outcomes for Children in Foster Care

Robin Mekonnen, MSW[a,b], Kathleen Noonan, JD[a],
David Rubin, MD, MSCE[a,c],*

KEYWORDS

- Foster care • Placement stability • Well being
- Health outcomes • Psychotropic medication
- Child welfare • System reform

In 2005, 513,000 children were living in foster homes in the United States. Several decades of research have demonstrated that nearly half of all children in foster care have chronic medical problems,[1–4] and up to 80% have serious emotional problems.[3,5–11] Despite the overwhelming evidence of need, studies consistently demonstrate that many health care needs of children in the foster care system go unmet. Stark evidence that children are not receiving timely services has come from a range of studies. The 1995 General Accounting Office report demonstrated that one third of children had health care needs that remained unaddressed while they were in out-of-home care, and a recent analysis of the National Survey of Child & Adolescent Well-Being documented that only a quarter of the children in out-of-home care who had behavioral problems received mental health services within a 1-year follow-up period.[12]

This article reviews the challenges health care systems have faced as they have attempted to improve health care outcomes for children in foster care. It discusses several of the promising health care strategies occurring outside the perimeter of child welfare and identifies some of the key impasses in working alongside efforts in child

This work was supported by a Stoneleigh Fellowship award and Grant No. 5K23HD045748 from the National Institute of Child Health & Development to D.R.

[a] PolicyLab: Center to Bridge Research, Practice and Policy at The Children's Hospital of Philadelphia, 34th and Civic Center Blvd., Philadelphia, PA 19104, USA
[b] School of Social Policy and Practice, The University of Pennsylvania, Philadelphia, PA, USA
[c] Department of Pediatrics, University of Pennsylvania School of Medicine, Philadelphia, PA, USA
* Corresponding author.
E-mail address: Rubin@email.chop.edu (D. Rubin).

welfare reform. The authors posit that the greatest impasse in establishing a reasonable quality of health care for these children is a child welfare practice and system in which children move frequently among multiple homes and in and out of the child welfare system. The central thesis of this article is to demonstrate the implausibility on improving health-related outcomes for children in foster care without fundamentally addressing the impact of frequent placement disruptions on the lives and well-being of children. Finally the authors propose potential strategies for targeting incremental reform efforts, specifically involving placement stability, as a vehicle for multidisciplinary reform inclusive of the health care system.

THE HEALTH CARE NEEDS OF CHILDREN IN FOSTER CARE: THE STATE OF THE STATE

Prior research establishing the large burden of unmet need among children in foster care has not been easy to reconcile with other data demonstrating the high intensity of service use by these children. Use of mental health services by children in foster care is 8 to 11 times greater than that experienced by other low-income and generally high-risk children in the Medicaid program.[13,14] Children in foster care account for 25% to 41% of mental health expenditures for children within the Medicaid program although they represent less than 3% of all enrollees.[14,15] The answer to this apparent contradiction lies in recent data showing that up to 90% of mental health costs may be accounted for by 10% of the children.[15,16] Because interventions often are difficult to acquire early on, the brunt of the services provided are being provided at the back end of the system, when children are living in residential treatment, group homes, psychiatric facilities, and hospital settings. A small number of children are receiving intensive, expensive services because the system has neglected them until their needs became catastrophic. This situation reflects a failure to screen adequately for behavioral health problems and to provide services to the overwhelming majority of children who otherwise could be excellent candidates for treatment and who probably would respond to more modest levels of treatment if such services were provided at the earliest possible time.

Ultimately, the failure to address the needs of children adequately while they are young and early in their placement into out-of-home care has manifested in poor long-term outcomes. Among former foster care youth in the Northwest Foster Care Alumni study from 2005, 54% reported at least one major mental health diagnosis, more than double the rate in the general population (22%). Foster care alumni reported almost three times the rate of anxiety disorders, twice the rate of depression, and four times the rate of substance abuse when compared with the general population. Most alarmingly, 25% reported symptoms of posttraumatic stress disorder, more than six times the rate in the general public and twice the rate experienced by returning war veterans (**Fig. 1**).[9]

THE ROLE OF PLACEMENT INSTABILITY IN EXACERBATING THE CRISIS

Although it would be easy to blame the poor health outcomes of children on the failure of public health systems to provide adequate settings to address the needs of these children, such a conclusion fails to consider the tremendous difficulty that disruptions in placement have on the ability to provide high-quality care. That is not to say that the health care system is absolved of fault in this discussion, but rather that a cascading relationship between disruptions in placement and worsening health outcomes has taxed the health care system. Placement disruptions exacerbate behavioral and other health problems among children, and they also make it more difficult to provide access to optimal care. For example, not only do caregivers change with every change

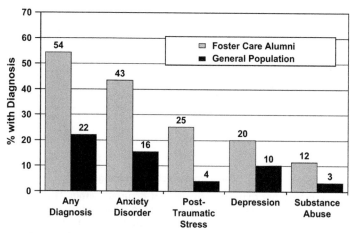

Fig. 1. The Northwest Alumni Study. (*From* Pecora PJ, Kessler RC, Williams J, et al. Improving family foster care: findings from the Northwest Foster Care Alumni Study. Seattle (WA): Casey Family Programs; 2005; with permission.)

in placement, but the often children also cycle through multiple health providers, each unaware of the child's past medical history and uncertain of the care plans for the child's medical and behavioral health problems. Changes in placement can thus prevent the establishment of continuous relationships with health service providers, inhibiting a provider's ability to get to know the child and the child's complete health history. In turn, caregivers who have little information about new foster children often disproportionately seek services from emergency departments. It is not surprising, then, that 75% of emergency department visits within 3 weeks of a placement change occur in the period immediately following that placement change (**Fig. 2**).[17]

The increasing use of psychotropic drugs by children in foster care is a clear example of the challenge that health care providers encounter.[18,19] The General Accounting Office in Washington recently reported that nearly one in three states have identified the oversight of psychotropic medication use in state foster care populations as one of the most pressing issues facing their child welfare systems in the next 5 years.[20] A recent study from the National Survey of Child and Adolescent Well-Being documented that 13.5% of children in the child welfare system were using medication, two to three times the rate of other children in the community.[21] Examination of Medicaid records from the State of Texas in 2004 revealed that 43% of children in foster care were using three or more medications concomitantly, and 22% were duplicating medications within the same pharmacologic class.[22]

The increasing use of psychotropic medications by children in foster care can be linked directly to the fragmented system of care for these children and the inadequate resources for assessment and treatment. It can also be linked to multiple placement moves, lack of foster parent and caseworker training, limited provision of information to caregivers about a child's specific needs and available services, and insufficient collaboration between child welfare, health, and mental health systems.[23–26] In addition, children in foster care who have challenging behaviors are likely to be treated with psychotropic medications in lieu of addressing the issues of instability and failed attachments that may be at the root of these behaviors. In practical terms, mental health professionals might perceive the suitability and efficacy of alternative

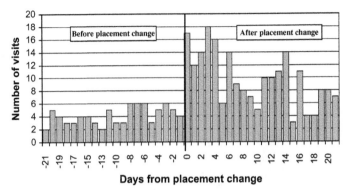

Fig. 2. Timing of emergency department visits that occurred within 21 days of entry into foster care or after placement changes for 2358 children entering foster care in Philadelphia from 1993 to 1996. (*From* Rubin D, Alessandrini E, Feudtner C, Localio A, Hadley T. Placement changes and emergency department visits in the first year of foster care. Pediatrics 2004;114(3):e354–60; with permission.)

behavioral interventions to be limited if children move frequently between homes or if they are likely to be under their professional care for only brief durations. Frequent moves between homes add the potential for treatment discontinuity that might expose children to the use of increasing numbers and combinations of medications, to their inappropriate administration, and even to abrupt discontinuation. Finally, children may lack an adult in their lives to consent and advocate for alternatives to medication when behavioral problems are identified. Of paramount concern is that placement instability can be linked directly to the failure to provide high-quality mental health treatment, and ultimately these failures affect children's duration of care, level of care, and opportunities for permanency.

Child Stability Issues Undermine the Potential Effectiveness of Several Promising Health Interventions

Several promising programs and practice models are seeking to improve the health care status of foster children. The "medical home" is one such model that recently was mandated in the Fostering Success Act of the 110th Congress that was signed into law by President Bush in October, 2008 (P.L. 110–351). The model advocates that children in foster care have a consistent "medical home" where the child maintains the same practitioner and receives all assessment and referrals for specialized care. The physicians in such settings also are able to influence case decisions and advocate to child welfare professionals in a more integrated fashion for possible interventions—be they in health or child welfare capacities—to improve the well being of the children they serve. The American Academy of Pediatrics Task Force on Health Care for Children in Foster Care has developed a set of standards defining the medical home model, emphasizing that care is comprehensive, coordinated, compassionate, consistent, culturally competent, and family focused.[27]

There are no data on the percentage of children in foster care who have a medical home. In the general population, the national median of all children who had medical homes was 47% percent, with a range among states from 33% to 61%.[28] It is probably a safe assumption that children in foster care fall far below any national median for participation in medical homes. The medical home model nonetheless holds promise as an optimal method for managing the complex medical needs of children in foster care. It also would provide an advocate to act on the child's behalf when issues of consent are raised for behavioral health treatments for children. Finally, by emphasizing continuity of care despite placement disruptions, a medical home can help prevent the loss of information about the child's health history and also can provide crisis management for the behavioral and physical health problems that so often escalate during this time period.[17]

Other promising approaches have been to provide more integrated models of care, whereby case management for health care services are co-located either virtually or physically with child welfare units. Many child welfare systems have taken advantage of the flexibility in case management funding within the Medicaid program to finance health care case management services within their agencies and have attempted to coordinate better the medical, educational, and social services for children in foster care. At least 38 states have used Medicaid targeted case management (TCM) funding in some capacity for their child welfare populations.[29] A 2005 Urban Institute study found that only about 17% of foster care children receive TCM; but those who do fare better in receiving health services than those without TCM.[30] For instance, 68% of children with TCM received physician services, versus 44% of children without TCM. Dental care (44% versus 24%), care from other practitioners (31% versus 14%), and therapy (11% versus 2%) are other vital health services that were obtained at greater rates among children with TCM.[30]

Many states and counties have used case management funding to create health care coordination units directly within their child welfare agencies. For some, this coordination has taken the form of health passports for children, using Medicaid claim data to create a medical history or profile for all of its recipients using a centralized database. Some states take this process one step further, and all Medicaid enrollees receive a smart card that contains a chip programmed with a summary of the child's medical history, including immunizations. Such a system offers the additional advantage of reducing the loss of medical information as a child moves in and out of the child welfare system.[31]

The State of Texas recently has invested heavily in developing a statewide health passport system for children entering foster care.[32] The record begins when the child is placed in out-of-home care and is updated and accessed via Web-based provider and caseworker access. The record is maintained only until the child exits care.[32] In the San Diego child welfare system, public health nurses monitor the health records of all children entering foster care, and data clerks assist in creating and maintaining a health passport (ie, a permanent transferable documentation of medical history) for children entering care but only while the children remain in care, similar to the Texas passport system.[33]

Other systems have focused less on the medical health passport and more on innovative strategies to improve access to and referral for mental health services. In Philadelphia, behavioral health workers are beginning to operate alongside intake workers for the child welfare system to triage and refer children who reportedly are exhibiting concerning behaviors. Other systems go much further by attempting to integrate newer models of mental health care delivery that partner the caregivers of children with mental health supports and services to improve health outcomes for children. The most cogent example of this approach is the multidimensional treatment foster care model, which operates as a more unrestricted placement for children in lieu of residential treatment. Caregivers more intensively trained for children who have behavioral problems serve a key role in this model, and in the best settings these caregivers are united with well-resourced supports and services that provide therapeutic services to children directly in their homes.[34,35]

Fundamental Challenges for Health Care Innovations

The programs discussed in the previous sections are only a few of many examples of the strategies that systems have invoked to coordinate the health care of children in foster care. A further discussion of other strategies can be found in the textbook authored by McCarthy,[36] *Meeting the Health Care Needs of Children in the Foster Care System.* Although these programs offer innovative approaches to addressing health disparities for children in foster care, the successful dissemination of these programs has often been problematic. Medical home models, for example, are easier to implement in smaller population centers, where a single center can provide a minimum standard of care for all children traversing the child welfare system, seeing children every time they change placement within a locality. In larger cities, where a single center is an implausible solution, and where children may move over large geographic distances when placements change, medical homes are less achievable. With regard to health passports, it remains uncertain who should fill out these passports, a problem that is magnified every time a child changes placement. Finally, with regard to integrated models of care such as treatment foster care, sustainable funding for case management is continuously threatened, most recently when the Deficit Reduction Act of 2005 sought to restrict the use of Medicaid funds for such purposes.[37]

Even when the financing is secure, the financial support required by integrated models can be both a boon for recruiting high-quality caregivers and a reverse incentive that actually can discourage caregivers from providing permanency to children. For instance, as the reimbursement for providing treatment-level foster care becomes more generous, it often exceeds what caregivers—and their agencies, for that matter—can receive in return for providing long-term permanency or adoption to children. Certainly, agencies will not want to lose their treatment-level caregivers to adoptions, given that the available pool of these caregivers is small, and the reverse can be true, also: treatment-level caregivers often wish to continue providing that level of care (with its reimbursement) and so are less likely to request adoptions. As a result, any gains realized in treatment foster care, such as improvements in child behavior, usually trigger another move for a step down in care. As such, gains often are lost when children are returned as a routine matter to more unrestricted settings with less support for behavioral issues and where the cascade of placement disruptions and poor outcomes can continue.

Certainly, the problems that continue to undermine the effectiveness of health innovations are not insurmountable. Some programs have tried to accommodate their models of care to minimize such problems. Chicago, for example, has developed an integrated network of health providers who receive enhanced Medicaid reimbursement and case management assistance to see children in foster care.[36] In addition, recent advances in information technology and cross-system data-sharing capacities may increase the potential for automating the completion of health passports through computer-generated abstraction of service claims, a solution that already is being invoked in some municipalities.

There is no lack of ingenuity and investment by health care professionals when it comes to developing promising approaches to address the complicated health needs of children in foster care. Each model's limitations, however, are amplified exponentially by the likelihood of disruption of placement and coverage and thus disruptions in continuity of care. Stability in placement is prerequisite for the success of practices that then can lead to better outcomes in health and well being for children in care over the long term.

System-Level Instability Also Undermines the Effectiveness of Health Innovations

At an organizational level, the instability in child welfare systems often mirrors the experience of children in their care, contributing to the problems in health and well being created by frequent and poorly monitored placement changes. In October, 2004 the Children's Bureau of the US Department of Health and Humans Services announced that none of the 50 states or United States territories was able to pass the first round of Children and Family Service Reviews.[38] Additionally no states achieved substantial conformity to the federal standards for placement stability.[39] At least 32 states and cities are operating pursuant to consent decrees, which are judgments entered into court by consent of both parties in which the defendant agrees to perform or stop performing specific activities; in most situations, the court maintains jurisdiction over the decree, requiring the parties to report regularly on the activities agreed to in the settlement document. Many of the decrees more than 10 years old, and 32 involve the provision of health services for children in foster care.[40] Under these circumstances, it is expected or mandated that radical transformations occur, but the track record of successful system change in these contexts has been mixed, at best.[41]

These system failings often result in mandates for procedural changes in an attempt to standardize practice through rules: add a new form here or an additional risk assessment there, as well as an abundance of "pilot" interventions or programs, many of which never get rolled out to system-wide implementation. In many child protective services agencies there is an order of what have been called "street-level bureaucrats," who use personal experience and discretion in managing case-level events[42] and who have seen multiple new projects come and go, offering little or no meaningful change in their daily operations. Front-line workers, who for the most part carry the burden of decision-making in foster-care cases, often do so with limited input from others and with very little routine supervision or accountability related to the quality of practice.[41,42]

Child welfare systems can present a revolving door of new agendas, new leaders, and new workers. At the leadership level, the average tenure of a child welfare director is about 2 years (T. Field, personal communication, 2008). New leaders commonly bring new agendas, and so the systems absorb that change as well. As for as front-line workers, research has demonstrated that caseworker turnover, which is estimated to be between 30% and 40% percent annually,[43] has a significant impact on child stability. When there is caseworker turnover and a new caregiver, in a field notorious for its incomplete and/or inaccurate case file documentation,[44] much of the child's past health or treatment history can be lost or unavailable in urgent circumstances.

Despite these challenges, system-level reform has occurred. Many leaders and advocates have recognized that years of myriad new procedures and mandates have created compliance-driven systems in which the clinical dimension of practice focuses on rules and deadlines and not on traditional family-centered social work. In many systems around the country, reforms now are attempting to create some stability by focusing on a consistent and basic skill set, sometimes referred to as the "practice model."[41] Importantly, these "practice model" reforms typically are combined with improvements in the system's ability to track performance through quantitative and qualitative data collection at the worker, provider, and system levels. These reforms hold some promise for greater stability and accountability in the child welfare system.

THE NEED FOR HEALTH INNOVATIONS ROOTED IN CHILD WELFARE REFORM

The enormous challenges of reducing placement instability for children and the more fundamental instability within child welfare systems may help explain why better health outcomes for children in foster care have been difficult to achieve. These challenges, however, do not relieve pediatricians of the responsibility of working for the required improvements in the system, whether in traditional and familiar areas of health care or in areas of financing and the delivery of child welfare services, where pediatricians rarely venture. What is needed, however, is a paradigm shift with respect to the expectations for and design of health care interventions in the context of the larger issue of the performance of the child welfare system. Indeed, the principal lesson learned in reviewing the history of health care delivery for children in foster care is that any health care intervention aimed at children in foster care needs to address the context of the system in which it will be housed. In other words, the road to more substantive reform in the delivery of quality health care to children in out-of-home placement starts with an actively engaged medical community participating in efforts to improve the child welfare system and to develop newer models that do not depend entirely on traditional health care providers (eg, in mental health) to fulfill the needs of these children.

Doctors and other health care providers who treat children in foster care must have a seat at the child welfare reform table. Their developmental perspective on issues such as placement stability could contribute enormously to system reform. Moreover, their opinion and expertise on issues such as how to respond to the trends around psychotropic drug use for children in foster care are critical. This kind of participation will require physicians to take a greater role in their own communities by providing oversight to the child welfare system and regular expert counsel to its leadership.

The goal of such an effort by physicians within the child welfare system would be to help create a permissive environment for health care reforms. To meet this goal, physicians must be advocates within their communities for efforts to reduce the size of the child welfare system and to improve placement stability and permanency for the children who will continue to need and depend on it. The best way to improve the efficacy of health interventions is to reduce the movement of children within the system and thereby make efforts in health care coordination more manageable. In addition to the mandatory reporting of suspected abuse, the physician may have an additional moral obligation to help a family identify practical alternatives to foster care, such as kinship caregivers who can facilitate a child's early exit from the system to permanency.[45] So physicians can be advocates for the families they report, even though mandatory reporting laws do not require physicians to identify placement alternatives nor are they responsible for the placement decisions that are made. At a systems level, physicians may need to advocate for more integrated, real-time surveillance and casework related to placement moves and for using stability, not simply adoption and reunification, as a metric to evaluate the performance of public and provider agencies. That call to action also would entail the responsibility of remaining engaged with child welfare systems and offering to participate in the monitoring of outcomes.

If systems become more manageable and children easier to track, many of the health care strategies discussed in this article will be more effective. Medical homes will be less likely to be disrupted and will serve as an extra check and balance in the system to make sure that adequate coordination is provided for children and that they remain safe in their homes. Health care passports will be easier to enforce and maintain. More efficient placement decisions made earlier in care also will translate to smaller populations of children needing to remain in supervised care, and for the children who do need supervised care, integrated models of care can be more narrowly directed, and the coordination of care will be easier to manage.

Finally, when the health problems for children in foster care are related to a fault of the health care system itself, such as in the poor availability of behavioral health providers for children, physicians can play a critical role in designing new interventions that rely less on physician involvement for consultation and more on training care-givers to be more adept in helping children who have significant behavioral problems. Much of this innovation is occurring already. Empiric family-based therapy aimed at empowering families to confront the behavioral needs of the their children more effec-tively is offering a promising approach to improving outcomes for children.[46] This promising approach is the ultimate realization that traditional health care options may have limited benefit for children in foster care, and that cross-disciplinary training and support will be more likely to succeed in the long term.

SUMMARY

Achieving better outcomes in health and well being for children in foster care will require contributions from a range of professional, community, and family networks. Physicians who treat children in foster care can play an important role in shaping better child welfare programs and policies on the basis of what is developmentally and medically best for children. An improved child welfare system will view child health and well-being outcomes, and the programs needed to achieve them, as central to its mission of care.

REFERENCES

1. US General Accounting Office. Foster care: health needs of many young children are unknown and unmet. Washington, DC: GAO/HEHS; 1995. p. 95–114.
2. Takayama J, Wolfe E, Coulter K. Relationship between reason for placement and medical findings among children in foster care. Pediatrics 1998;101(2): 201–7.
3. Halfon N, Mendonca A, Berkowitz G. Health status of children in foster care. The experience of the center for the vulnerable child. Arch Pediatr Adolesc Med 1995; 149(4):386–92.
4. Simms M. The foster care clinic: a community program to identify treatment needs of children in foster care. J Dev Behav Pediatr 1989;10(3):121–8.
5. Clausen J, Landsverk J, Ganger W, et al. Mental health problems of children in foster care. J Child Fam Stud 1998;7(3):283–96.
6. Garland A, Hough R, Landsverk J, et al. Racial and ethnic variations in mental health care utilization among children in foster care. Child Serv Soc Policy Res Pract 2000;3(3):133–46.
7. Glisson C. The effects of services coordination teams on outcomes for children in state custody. Adm Soc Work 1994;18:1–23.
8. Landsverk J, Garland A, Leslie L. Mental health services for children reported to child protective services, vol. 2. Thousand Oaks (CA): Sage Publications; 2002.
9. Pecora P, Kessler R, Williams J, et al. Improving family foster care: findings from the Northwest Foster Care Alumni Study. Seattle (WA): Casey Family Programs; 2005. Available at: http://www.casey.org. Accessed February 2009.
10. Trupin E, Tarico V, Low B, et al. Children on child protective service caseloads: prevalence and nature of serious emotional disturbance. Child Abuse Negl 1993;17(3):345–55.

11. Urquiza A, Wirtz S, Peterson M, et al. Screening and evaluating abused and neglected children entering protective custody. Child Welfare 1994;73(2):155–71.

12. Burns B, Phillips S, Wagner R, et al. Mental health need and access to mental health services by youths involved with child welfare: a national survey. J Am Acad Child Adolesc Psychiatry 2004;43(8):960–70.

13. Harman J, Childs G, Kelleher K. Mental health care utilization and expenditures by children in foster care [see comments]. Arch Pediatr Adolesc Med 2000; 154(11):1114–7.

14. Halfon N, Berkowitz G, Klee L. Children in foster care in California: an examination of Medicaid reimbursed health services utilization. Pediatrics 1992;89(6 Pt 2):1230–7.

15. Takayama J, Bergman A, Connell F. Children in foster care in the state of Washington. Health care utilization and expenditures. JAMA 1994;271(23):1850–5.

16. Rubin D, Alessandrini E, Feudtner C, et al. Placement stability and mental health costs for children in foster care. Pediatrics 2004;113(5):1336–41.

17. Rubin D, Alessandrini E, Feudtner C, et al. Placement changes and emergency department visits in the first year of foster care. Pediatrics 2004;114(3):e354–60.

18. Olfson M, Blanco C, Liu L, et al. National trends in the outpatient treatment of children and adolescents with antipsychotic drugs. Arch Gen Psychiatry 2006;63(6):679–85.

19. Carey B. Use of antipsychotics by the Young Rose Fivefold. New York Times, June 6, 2006.

20. US Government Accountability Office. Child welfare: improving social service programs, training, and technical assistance information would help address long-standing service-level and workforce challenges. Washington, DC: US GAO; 2006. GAO-07-75.

21. Raghavan R, Zima B, Andersen R, et al. Psychotropic medication use in a national probability sample of children in the child welfare system. J Child Adolesc Psychopharmacol 2005;15(1):97–106.

22. Zito J, Safer D, Sai D, et al. Psychotropic medication patterns among youth in foster care. Pediatrics 2008;121(1):e157–63.

23. Garland A, Landsverk J, Lau A. Racial/ethnic disparities in mental health service use among children in foster care. Child Youth Serv Rev 2003;25(5/6):491–507.

24. Leslie L, Hurlburt M, Landsverk J, et al. Outpatient mental health services for children in foster care: a national perspective. Child Abuse Negl 2004;28(6):697–712.

25. Molin R, Palmer S. Consent and participation: ethical issues in the treatment of children in out-of-home care. Am J Orthop 2005;75(1):152–7.

26. Rubin D, Hafner L, Luan X, et al. Placement stability and early behavioral outcomes for children in out-of-home care. Paper presented at Child Protection: Using Research to Improve Policy and Practice, Washington, DC 2005.

27. Task Force on Health Care for Children in Foster Care. Fostering health: health care for children and adolescents in foster care. 2nd edition. Elk Grove Village (IL): American Academy of Pediatrics; 2005.

28. Shea K, Davis K, Schor E. U.S. variations in child health system performance: a state scorecard. New York: The Commonwealth Fund; 2008.

29. First Focus. Addressing the health care needs of foster care children. May 2008. Available at: http://www.firstfocus.net/Download/FosterCareHealth.pdf. Accessed February 2009.

30. Geen R, Sommers A, Cohen M. Medicaid spending on foster children. Washington, DC: Urban Institute; 2005.

31. Pindus N, Koralek R, Bernstein J, et al. The health passport project: assessment and recommendations-executive summary. Washington, DC: Urban Institute; 2001.

32. Texas Health and Human Services. Available at: http://www.hhs.state.tx.us/medicaid/FosterCare_FAQ.shtml. Accessed October 1, 2008.
33. Child Health and Disability Prevention (CHDP) Foster Care program. (Site Visit Report). San Diego County (CA): Georgetown University Child Development Center; 2000.
34. Fisher P, Kim H. Intervention effects on foster preschoolers' attachment-related behaviors from a randomized trial. Prev Sci 2007;8:161–70.
35. Price J, Chamberlain P, Landsverk J, et al. Effects of a foster parent training intervention on placement changes of children in foster care. Child Maltreat 2008;13:64–75.
36. McCarthy J. Meeting the health care needs of children in the foster care system. Washington, DC: Georgetown University; 2002.
37. Rubin D, Halfon N, Raghavan R, et al. The Deficit Reduction Act of 2005: implications for children receiving child welfare services. Washington, DC: Casey Family Programs; 2006.
38. U.S. Department of Health and Human Services. Child and Family Services reviews update. Washington, DC: U.S. Department of Health and Human Services; 2004.
39. U.S. Department of Health and Human Services. General findings from the federal child and family services review: 2001–2004. Available at: http://www.acf.hhs.gov/programs/cb/cwmonitoring/results/genfindings04/index.htm. Accessed February 2009.
40. Child welfare consent decrees: analysis of thirty-five court actions from 1995–2005. Washington, DC: Child Welfare League of America, National Child Welfare Resource Center on Legal and Judicial Issues; 2005.
41. Noonan K, Sabel C, Simon W. Legal accountability in the service-based welfare state: lessons from child welfare reform. Law Soc Inq 2009, in press.
42. Lipsky M. Street level bureaucracy: dilemmas of the individual in public services. New York: Russell Sage Foundation; 1980.
43. HHS could play a greater role in helping child welfare agencies recruit and retain staff. Washington, DC: U.S. General Accounting Office; 2003.
44. Gelles R. Book of David: how preserving families can cost children's lives. Basic Books; 1997.
45. Rubin D, Downes K, O'Reilly A, et al. Impact of kinship care on behavioral well-being for children in out-of-home care. Arch Pediatr Adolesc Med 2008;162:550–6.
46. Barth R, Landsverk J, Chamberlain P, et al. Parent training in child welfare services: planning for a more evidence-based approach to serving biological parents. Res Soc Work Pract 2005;15(5):353–71.

Mental Health Treatment of Child Abuse and Neglect: The Promise of Evidence-Based Practice

Kimberly Shipman, PhD*, Heather Taussig, PhD

KEYWORDS

- Child abuse • Mental health treatment
- Evidence-based practice • Child trauma • Child maltreatment

In 2006, 3.6 million children in the United States received a child protective services' investigation and 905,000 children (about one-quarter of those investigated) were found to have been abused and/or neglected.[1] The majority of maltreated youth had substantiated neglect (64.1%), followed by physical abuse (16.0%), sexual abuse (8.8%), psychological maltreatment (6.6%) and other types (15.1%) (nonexclusive categories). There was fairly equal gender distribution among the child victims, with 51.5% of the victims being female. Younger children had higher rates of maltreatment than older children; African American and American Indian/Alaskan Native children were overrepresented among children substantiated for maltreatment.[1] In 2006, 303,000 children entered out-of-home care (including foster care, kinship care, residential treatment, group homes) and 510,000 children were in care on September 30, 2006. African American children and multiracial children were overrepresented among children in care.[2]

Children who have been maltreated are at risk for experiencing a host of mental health problems including depression, post-traumatic stress, dissociation, reactive

The first author would like to acknowledge support from the Substance Abuse and Mental Health Services Administration (5 SM058184-02, K. Shipman, PI) for this project. The second author would like to acknowledge support from National Institute for Mental Health (R01 MH076919 (H. Taussig, PI). We would also like to acknowledge support from the Kempe Foundation.
University of Colorado, School of Medicine, The Kempe Center for the Prevention and Treatment of Child Abuse and Neglect, The Gary Pavillion at the Children's Hospital, Anschutz Medical Campus, 13123 East 16th Avenue, Box B390, Aurora, CO 80045, USA
* Corresponding author.
E-mail address: shipman.kimberly@tchden.org (K. Shipman).

Pediatr Clin N Am 56 (2009) 417–428
doi:10.1016/j.pcl.2009.02.002
0031-3955/09/$ – see front matter © 2009 Published by Elsevier Inc.

pediatric.theclinics.com

attachment, low self-esteem, social problems, suicidal behavior, aggression, conduct disorder, attention-deficit hyperactivity disorder (ADHD) and problem behaviors, including delinquency, risky sexual behavior and substance use.[3–6] In a sample of 426 children receiving child welfare services, 42% met diagnostic criteria for a DSM-IV diagnosis based on youth- and parent-report.[5] ADHD and Disruptive Disorders, such as Oppositional Defiant Disorder and Conduct Disorder, were among the diagnoses most frequently assigned to youth in the child welfare system.[5,7] Not surprisingly, maltreated children who are placed in out-of-home care also manifest a host of emotional, behavioral, social and developmental problems, and they are in need of many specialized services.[8,9] Based on their review of the epidemiologic literature describing the mental health needs of youth in out-of-home care, Landsverk and Garland[9] reported that "between one-half and two-thirds of the children entering foster care exhibit behavior or social competency problems warranting mental health services." Studies of Medicaid claims suggest that as many as 57% of youth in foster care meet Medicaid criteria for a mental disorder.[10]

Given the high rate of mental health problems, it is not surprising that maltreated youth are in need of mental health services. Unfortunately, only a fraction of these children and adolescents receive services. For example, in one nationally representative study, between 37%–44% of youth with child welfare service involvement scored in the borderline or clinical ranges on parent-, teacher- and self-report measures of mental health and behavioral functioning; only 11% of these youth, however, were receiving outpatient mental health services.[6] Rates of service use are higher among children placed in out-of-home care.[11] One study found that children in foster care in California, who comprised less than 4% of Medi-Cal-eligible children, accounted for 41% of all users of Medi-Cal mental health services.[12] Another study found that children in foster care used more mental health services (including hospitalizations), at greater expense than children in the Aid to Families with Dependent Children (AFDC) program or children receiving Supplemental Security Income (SSI).[7,10] Despite reported high rates of service use of children in foster care, many youth in out-of-home care also do not receive needed services.[13] For example, one study found that 80% of children ages 6–12 in foster care were given a psychiatric diagnosis, yet only 50% had received mental health or special education services[14] and another study found that only 23% of children in foster care had received some type of mental health service.[13]

Exacerbating the problem of effectively treating mental health problems in maltreated youth is the lack of evidence-based mental health treatment available, even for those children and adolescents who do receive treatment. The tide may be turning for our most vulnerable youth, however. Recently, several evidence-based practices have been rigorously tested and are demonstrating efficacy in reducing mental health problems associated with maltreatment.

WHAT IS EVIDENCE-BASED PRACTICE?

There has been a recent surge in interest in identifying, evaluating, and disseminating evidence-based practices for child abuse and neglect.[15–17] Evidence-based practice (EBP) can be defined simply as using clinical interventions that have the best scientific support for their effectiveness. EBP typically have well-developed treatment manuals, established training protocols for clinicians, and ongoing assessment of clinician fidelity to the treatment model. EBP is unique from more traditional practice given that treatment effectiveness is demonstrated incrementally through well-designed, randomized clinical trials using outcomes that are tied to specific treatment goals.

Early clinical trials are typically conducted in controlled settings to determine treatment efficacy or the ability of the treatment to yield effects under ideal circumstances. After efficacy has been established, effectiveness trials are conducted to determine if the model will work when put into practice more widely within community-based settings. A scientific approach to determining treatment effectiveness avoids the many pitfalls that are encountered when relying on case studies or nonrandomized group comparisons, clinician judgement of progress, or outcomes that are not directly related to intervention goals (eg, client satisfaction) (See Chafin[15] for a detailed discussion). It is important to note that EBP also shares many characteristics with traditional practice, including the recognition of the importance of core nonspecific factors (eg, client–therapist relationship), clinician interpersonal skills, and common codes of good practice and professional ethics.

IDENTIFYING EVIDENCE-BASED PRACTICES FOR MALTREATED CHILDREN

Two recent projects have focused on identifying EBP for treating abused children and their families. In 2003, a project funded by the U.S. Office for Victims of Crime (OVC) developed guidelines for treatment of child physical and sexual abuse.[18] The primary goal of this project was to provide information to clinicians to encourage the use of theoretically-sound, empirically-based interventions for child abuse. To develop these guidelines, a national advisory group was convened to establish criteria to rate the extent of support available for 24 interventions that addressed concerns associated with child physical and sexual abuse. Criteria included the strength of empiric support, soundness of theoretical foundation, potential for harm, clinical utility, and acceptance among clinicians. Ratings ranged from the highest rating of "well-supported and efficacious" to the lowest rating of "concerning treatment." Trauma-focused Cognitive Behavioral Therapy (TF-CBT)[19] was the only intervention that received the highest rating. Fifteen of the remaining interventions, however, were rated as "supported and probably efficacious" or "supported and acceptable."

The Kauffman Best Practices Project[20] followed up on the OVG guideline project to systematically identify a small number of best practice interventions from the 24 already identified. The primary goal was to increase dissemination and use of these best practices among clinicians treating abused children and their families. The project convened a broad range of advisors including researchers, treatment providers, managers of clinical programs, and representatives from Authentic Voices International, an organization of adult, child abuse survivors dedicated to helping others recover from child abuse trauma. The advisory group identified three best practices based on criteria that emphasized research support, clinical acceptability, and the transportability to typical clinical settings. The three best practices identified were TF-CBT,[10] Parent-Child Interaction Therapy (PCIT),[21,22] and Abuse-Focused-Cognitive Behavioral Therapy (AF-CBT).[23] (As the authors note, these are not the only interventions that could have been identified as best practices. These interventions, however, did have the greatest level of theoretical, empiric, and clinical support and consensus among committee members.)

The National Child Traumatic Stress Network (NCTSN) is also an excellent resource for identifying evidence-based practices in child abuse and neglect. NCTSN is a unique collaboration of academic and community-based service centers from all over the United States whose mission is to raise the standard of care and to increase access to evidence-based services for traumatized children and their families, including children exposed to child abuse. Through considerable interagency collaboration, NCTSN has identified evidence-based and promising practices for child trauma and has developed strategies for effective dissemination of these interventions. The NCTSN Web site (www.nctsn.org) has considerable information about EBP as well as about other resources helpful to medical, mental health, and child welfare professionals. This Web site also has a list of grantees from all over the United States who can provide information regarding treatment referrals in their communities.

EVIDENCE-BASED PRACTICES FOR CHILD MALTREATMENT

The goal of this section is to highlight some of the most promising EBP in the treatment of child maltreatment. It is important to note that this is not an exhaustive list of well-supported interventions. Information about other evidence-based and promising practices for child abuse and neglect can be found in the resources discussed above (www.nctsn.org),[18,20] as well as in recently published literature reviews on this topic.[17,19]

Parenting Interventions

Parent–child interaction therapy

PCIT is a short-term, behavioral intervention for children and their parents that is focused on enhancing the quality of the parent–child relationship and teaching positive approaches to child behavior management.[21,22] PCIT was originally developed to treat children 2 to 7 years of age with behavioral problems, but it has recently been adapted for physically abusive parents and their children up to age 12.[24] PCIT has two primary treatment components. The first component focuses on teaching parents relationship-building skills (ie, praise, reflection, imitation, description, enthusiasm) through a combination of didactic training and coaching of parent–child interaction. The second component uses didactic training and coaching of parent–child interaction to teach skills central to positive behavior management (eg, effective use of commands, strategies for increasing compliance). Numerous clinical trials have demonstrated the efficacy of PCIT in reducing child behavior problems and parent–child interaction problems in a variety of populations.[25–27] Treatment effects have been demonstrated to maintain over time[27,28] and to generalize to untreated siblings[29] and to school settings.[30] A recent randomized clinical trial with physically maltreating families[24] indicates that PCIT substantially reduced the re-report rate for physical abuse as compared with a standard community-based parenting group (19% re-report rate for PCIT group; 49% for standard care group at a median follow-up of 850 days post-treatment). The superiority of PCIT was mediated by a greater reduction in negative parenting behaviors in the PCIT group. PCIT has been used clinically with diverse populations, with cultural adaptations available for Mexican Americans and Native American families.[31] Preliminary research, based on uncontrolled, pre/post-test designs, suggests that PCIT shows promise for treating children in foster care[32] and for training foster parents.[33]

Abuse-focused cognitive behavioral therapy

Abuse-focused cognitive behaviorial therapy (AF-CBT)[23] is a short-term intervention for physically abusive parents and their school-age children based on behavioral, cognitive-behavioral, and family systems theories. Treatment delivery is organized into three phases, which include: psychoeducation and engagement; individual and family skills training; and family applications. Core components include development of: (a) child-directed skills (eg, psychoeducation about abuse; cognitive processing of abuse-related experiences; emotion regulation and coping skills; social support planning); (b) parent-directed skills (eg, understanding coercive behavior; processing/challenging views on hostility, child-related developmental expectations, and maladaptive attributions; emotion regulation; positive approaches to discipline); and (c) parent–child or family system components (eg, safety planning; no violence agreement; clarification to establish responsibility for abuse and focus on needs of victim/family; family problem-solving and communication skills). In a small, randomized clinical trial, the individual (parent and child components) and family approaches in AF-CBT were compared, respectively, to routine community services. Findings demonstrated that both the individual and the family components resulted in greater reduction in children's externalizing problems, child-to-parent violence, parental distress and abuse risk, and family conflict and cohesion.[34] AF-CBT has been used clinically with urban African American families and has been reviewed by African American stakeholders for relevance and clinical utility.

Interventions for Child Trauma

Trauma-focused cognitive behavioral therapy
TF-CBT[19,35,36] is a short-term, cognitive-behavioral intervention used to treat traumatized children ages 3 to 17. Although TF-CBT was originally developed for child sexual abuse, this model has been used to treat children exposed to multiple types of trauma.[37] Core treatment components include: psycho-education about trauma; strategies for managing distressing feelings, thoughts and behavior; exposure to and processing of trauma-related memories through development of a trauma narrative; and enhancing parenting skills and child safety. Children and non-offending parents are initially seen individually but, when ready, come together so that the child may share the trauma narrative with his or her parent. A number of randomized clinical trials have demonstrated the superiority of TF-CBT over nondirective play therapy and child-centered therapies in traumatized children with regard to several areas of child functioning (eg, posttraumatic stress symptoms, anxiety, depression, externalizing behaviors, sexualized behaviors, shame)[19] (see Cohen et al for a review). Additionally, parents who participate in treatment show improvements with regard to parenting practices and the ability to support their child as well as reductions in their own levels of depression and distress about their child's abuse. Treatment gains are maintained at one-and two-year follow-up.[38–40] TF-CBT has been used with diverse populations (eg, African American, Latino) and with children in foster care.

Child–parent psychotherapy
Child–parent psychotherapy (CPP)[41] is an attachment-based intervention used to treat traumatized children from birth to six years of age. CPP emphasizes the importance of treating mental health problems from within the context of the parent-child relationship by working with the parent-child dyad. Treatment targets several areas including safety, affect regulation, and the quality of the child-parent relationship as well as joint processing of child's trauma experiences. Typical treatment duration is 50 sessions. Randomized, clinical trials with maltreated children have indicated the superiority of CPP over standard community services with regard to enhancing the quality of the parent-child attachment relationship[42] and the child's representations of self and caregivers.[43] A third randomized trial demonstrated that CPP, as compared with a case management/individual psychotherapy group, resulted in greater reductions in behavioral problems and traumatic stress symptoms in children who had witnessed domestic violence and greater reductions in parent's avoidance PTSD symptoms.[44] Additionally, gains in child and maternal functioning were maintained at 6 month follow-up.[45] Related clinical trial research has demonstrated the efficacy of CPP with regard to improvements in the quality of the parent–child relationship as indicated by attachment security and both parent (ie, increased empathy and interactiveness with children) and child behaviors (eg, decreased anger, avoidance,

resistance, increased partnership with mother) in different clinical groups (ie, anxiously attached children of recent immigrants; maternal depression).[46,47] Clinical trials were conducted with predominantly ethnic minority samples and CPP has been used clinically with many diverse groups (ie, Mexican, Central and South American, African American, and Chinese).

Interventions for Children in Out-of-Home Care

Although children placed in foster care are at substantial risk for a host of mental health problems and a number of adverse life outcomes, these findings do not necessarily suggest that foster care, per se, causes or contributes to these outcomes. In fact, we have found that maltreated children who were placed and remained in foster care demonstrated better functioning than maltreated children who reunified with their biologic families or maltreated children who were never removed from their homes.[48,49] The sequelae of maltreatment, described above, likely contribute to the identified problems for foster youth. Studies that have interviewed youth currently and formerly placed in foster care report that youth generally have positive feelings about foster care. Most thought placement was necessary and in their best interests, and they reported that things would have gotten worse at home without child welfare intervention.[50–53]

Although foster care placement is, in most cases, a necessary intervention, children in foster care are still at significant risk for adverse mental health outcomes, as they suffer the consequences of child maltreatment and experience additional trauma when they are removed and often isolated from their homes, schools, friends and families. Furthermore, these stressors may be exacerbated by placement changes. In addition to their already increased risk of emotional and behavioral problems, many of these youth lack appropriate coping resources to handle the multiplicity of stressors associated with multiple life transitions.[12,54]

There are significant challenges in developing and implementing evidence-based mental health treatments for youth in foster care. Conducting randomized controlled trials with a population in which custody and placements change frequently can lead to low recruitment rates and high attrition. Not surprisingly, then, there have been only a few studies of evidence-based practices that have been rigorously tested in foster care populations.

Multidimensional treatment foster care

One of the most well-regarded treatments for the reduction of significant behavior problems among adolescents is Multidimensional Treatment Foster Care (MTFC). Until recently, however, MTFC had not been tested with maltreated populations who had been placed into out-of-home care, because it was focused on adjudicated delinquent populations. A recent, randomized controlled trial was conducted in San Diego, CA. Keeping Foster Parents Trained and Supported (KEEP) was an effectiveness trial of a modification of MTFC conducted with 700 foster and kinship families who were caring for children, ages 5–12 years old, placed in out-of-home care through social services. The modified MTFC intervention consisted of 16 weeks of a 90-minute parent management group (traditional MTFC services include several additional components that were not implemented in this trial), consisting of 3–10 foster parents. Groups employed didactic presentations, group discussions, role playing, and videos to help foster parents increase their use of positive reinforcement and reduce their use of discipline. It also focused on teaching foster parents to use non-harsh discipline. Similar to findings with delinquent populations, the effectiveness trial reduced behavior problems for children in the treatment condition. These effects were concentrated among children with high levels of initial behavior problems and the effect was mediated by parenting practices.[55]

Early intervention foster care

Early Intervention Foster Care (EIFC) is a modification of MTFC for preschool-age (ages 3–6) maltreated children who have been placed in out-of-home care. Specialized foster parents receive training before children being placed in their homes. After children are placed, they receive ongoing support from program staff. Biologic parents also receive training if the permanency plan is for children to reunify. In addition to parent training, the intervention also includes a therapeutic playgroup and services provided by a behavioral specialist who works with families in their homes. Similar to MTFC, parents are encouraged to provide more reinforcement than discipline and to provide a predictable routine that enhances the development of children in their care. In a small, quasi-experimental study with 30 parent–child dyads, parenting practices improved, children evidenced better behavioral functioning, and there was a reduction in salivary cortisol over time in the intervention group, which the authors attributed to reduced stress.[56] A randomized controlled trial of the EIFC program was subsequently conducted with 90 children and families. This study demonstrated fewer failed permanent placements for children in the intervention arm.[57]

Attachment and biobehavioral catch-up

Attachment and Biobehavioral Catch-up (ABC) is a 10-week parent–child intervention aimed at enhancing regulatory capabilities in infants and young children. The intervention focuses on training foster parents to nurture the children in their care by: (1) following their child's lead; (2) engaging in positive physical touching (eg, hugging); and (3) allowing children to express emotions. In this study, 60 foster parent–child dyads (ages 3 to 39 months) were randomized to receive ether an educational intervention or the ABC intervention. One month after completion of the intervention, children in the treatment group evidenced better regulatory capability, as measured by a more typical pattern of cortisol production. There was no significant difference in parent-reported behavior problems in the two experimental groups.[58]

Incredible years adaptation

The Incredible Years (IY) is an evidence-based parenting program for children ages 3–10 years who are at risk of developing conduct disorder. The intervention was adapted for use with a foster care sample, in which foster and biologic parent pairs received the IY intervention together, along with a coparenting component, aimed at increasing positive parenting practices and ultimately reducing child behavior problems. The study randomly assigned 64 foster and biologic parent pairs to the intervention condition or treatment as usual. The intervention group received 12 weeks of manualized groups, which included 4 components (ie, play, praise and rewards, effective limit setting, and handling misbehavior) that were taught through videos, role playing, and homework. The coparenting component was delivered to the parent dyads in separate sessions and included opportunities to practice effective communication and resolve conflict. The intervention group demonstrated gains in positive parenting, and improvements in coparenting (only immediately following the intervention), and there was a trend for fewer externalizing behaviors among children in the intervention.[59]

Wraparound services

In an innovative study, 132 children in foster care (ages 7–15 years) with behavioral and/or emotional disturbances were randomized to either a services-as-usual condition or a "wraparound" services condition. The wraparound services consisted of "individualized, case-managed, collaborative" services that were implemented by family specialists. The four components of the services provided by the family specialists included strength-based assessment, life-domain planning, clinical case management, and follow-along supports and services. Children who received these enhanced services demonstrated greater improvement in emotional and behavioral adjustment over time according to their caregivers (there was no difference based on youth self-reports).[60]

Fostering healthy futures

Fostering Healthy Futures (FHF) is an ongoing randomized, controlled trial of a novel intervention for preadolescent youth in out-of-home care. The intervention consists of three components. First, all youth receive a no-cost evaluation of their mental health, cognitive functioning, and academic achievement. The findings are summarized in a screening report that is given to their caseworkers. After the baseline assessment has been completed, approximately one half of the youth are randomized to the prevention program, FHF. Children in the prevention arm of the trial receive a 30-week therapeutic skills group and one-on-one mentoring from graduate students in social work.[61] Thus far, FHF has enrolled 261 children into this innovative program and it has high rates of recruitment and retention (over 90% at each time point). Outcomes are expected to be published in the upcoming year.

FUTURE DIRECTIONS

Recent research in EBP for child maltreatment is exciting and has already had a significant impact on enhancing the quality of mental health services for maltreated children and their families. This work, however, is still in its infancy. Additional efficacy research is needed to expand the understanding of existing evidence-based practices and to evaluate other promising intervention programs. Specific goals for ongoing efficacy research would include: addressing methodological challenges common in this research (eg, small sample size, low retention rates); evaluating intervention appropriateness for diverse populations; and developing effective strategies to enhance already promising and efficacious interventions. Research should also focus on adapting and evaluating current EBP for use with additional types of trauma, different developmental levels, and comorbid conditions.[19] Children who are neglected constitute one population that needs particular attention given the paucity of research on treatment efficacy. The SafeCare Program[62] is a promising intervention that directly addresses problems associated with child neglect as well as child maltreatment more generally. Preliminary support based on nonrandomized research trials suggests that the SafeCare Program, as compared with standard community services, significantly reduces recurrence of child maltreatment (including neglect) and enhances positive parenting behaviors. Finally, there is a need to develop and evaluate strategies for effective dissemination and implementation of EBP in the community context. Work in this area must address challenges to the adoption of EBP at community, organizational, and clinician levels, which will require considerable collaboration among researchers, community mental health agencies, and child welfare.

REFERENCES

1. US Department of Health & Human Services. Administration on children, youth and families. In child maltreatment 2006. Chapter3. Available at: http://www.acf.hhs.gov/programs/cb/pubs/cm06/chapter3.htm. Accessed on: September 10, 2008.

2. US Department of Health & Human Services. Administration on children, youth and families. The AFCARS report preliminary FY 2006 estimates as of January 2008. Available at: http://www.acf.hhs.gov/programs/cb/stats_research/afcars/tar/report14.htm. Accessed on: September 10, 2008.

3. Briere J, Berliner L, Bulkley JA, et al. The APSAC handbook on child maltreatment. Thousand Oaks, CA: Sage Publications, Inc; 1996.

4. Welfare Information Gateway Child. Long-term consequences of child abuse and neglect. Available at: http://www.childwelfare.gov/pubs/factsheets/long_term_consequences.cfm. Accessed on: April 2008.

5. Garland AF, Hough RL, McCabe KM, et al. Prevalence of psychiatric disorders in youths across five sectors of care. J Am Acad Child Adolesc Psychiatry 2001;40(4):409–18.

6. National Survey of Child and Adolescent Well-Being. NSCAW one year in foster care wave 1 data analysis report, executive summary. Available at: http://www.acf.hhs.gov/programs/opre/abuse_neglect/nscaw/reports/exesum_nscaw/exsum_nscaw.pdf. Accessed October 28, 2008.

7. Harman JS, Childs GE, Kelleher KJ. Mental health care utilization and expenditures by children in foster care. Arch Pediatr Adolesc Med 2000;154:1114–7.

8. Clausen JM, Landsverk J, Ganger W, et al. Mental health problems of children in foster care. J Child Fam Stud 1998;7(3):283–96.

9. Landsverk J, Garland A. Foster care and pathways to mental health services. In: Curtis P, Dale G Jr, editors. The foster care crisis: translating research into practice and policy. Nebraska: The University of Nebraska Press; 1998. p. 193–210.

10. dosReis S, Zito JM, Safer DJ, et al. Mental health services for youths in foster care and disabled youths. Am J Public Health 2001;91(7):1094–9.

11. National Survey of Child and Adolescent Well-Being. NSCAW No. 3: children's cognitive and socioemotional development and their receipt of special educational and mental health services, research brief, findings from the NSCAW study. Available at: http://www.acf.hhs.gov/programs/opre/abuse_neglect/nscaw/reports/spec_education/spec_education.pdf. Accessed October 28, 2008.

12. Halfon N, Berkowitz G, Klee L. Mental health service utilization by children in foster care in California. Pediatrics 1992;89(6):1238–44.

13. National Survey of Child and Adolescent Well-Being. NSCAW one year in foster care wave 1 data analysis report. Available at:http://www.acf.hhs.gov/programs/opre/abuse_neglect/nscaw/reports/nscaw_oyfc/oyfc_report.pdf. Accessed October 28, 2008.

14. Zima BT, Bussing R, Yang X. Help-seeking steps and service use for children in foster care. J Behav Health Serv Res 2000;27(3):271–85.

15. Chaffin M, Friedrich W. Evidence-based treatments in child abuse and neglect. Child Youth Serv Rev 2004;26:1097–113.

16. Cohen JA, Mannarino AP, Murray LK, et al. Psychosocial interventions for maltreated and violence-exposed children. J Soc Issues 2006;62(4):737–66.

17. Silverman WK, Ortiz CD, Viswesvaran C, et al. Evidence-based psychosocial treatments for children and adolescents exposed to traumatic events. J Clin Child Adolesc Psychol 2008;37(1):156–83.

18. Saunders BE, Berliner L, Hanson RF. Child physical and sexual abuse: guidelines for treatment. Charleston, SC: National Crime Victims and Treatment Center; 2003 (Final Report: January 15, 2003).

19. Cohen JA, Mannarino AP, Deblinger E. Treating trauma and traumatic grief in children and adolescents. New York: Guilford Press; 2006.

20. Chadwick Center on Children and Families. Closing the quality chasm in child abuse treatment: identifying and disseminating best practices. San Diego, CA: Author; 2004.
21. Eyberg SM, Boggs SR. Parent-child interaction therapy: a psychosocial intervention for the treatment of young conduct disordered children. In: Schaefer CE, Briesmeister JM, editors. Handbook of parent training: Parents as co-therapists for children's behavior problems. 2nd edition. New York: John Wiley & Sons; 1998. p. 61–97.
22. Hembree-Kigin TL, McNeil C. Parent-child interaction therapy. New York: Plenum; 1995.
23. Kolko DJ, Swenson C. Assessing and treating physically abused children and their families: a cognitive behavioral approach. Thousand Oaks, CA: Sage Publications; 2002.
24. Chaffin M, Silovsky JF, Funderburk B, et al. Parent-child interaction therapy with physically abusive parents: efficacy for reducing future abuse reports. J Consult Clin Psychol 2004;72(3):500–10.
25. Bagner DM, Eyberg SM. Parent-child interaction therapy for disruptive behavior in children with mental retardation: a randomized controlled trial. J Clin Child Adolesc Psychol 2007;36(3):418–29.
26. Nixon RD, Sweeny L, Erickson DB, et al. Parent-child interaction therapy: a comparison of standard and abbreviated treatments for oppositional defiant preschoolers. J Consult Clin Psycho 2003;71(2):251–60.
27. Schuhmann EM, Foote RC, Eyberg SM, et al. Efficacy of parent-child interaction therapy: interim report of a randomized trial with short-term maintenance. J Clin Child Psychol 1998;27:34–45.
28. Hood KK, Eyberg SM. Outcomes of parent-child interaction therapy: mothers' reports of maintenance three to six years after treatment. J Clin Child Adolesc Psychol 2003;32(3):419–29.
29. Brestan EV, Eyberg SM, Boggs SR, et al. Parent-child interaction therapy: parents' perceptions of untreated siblings. Child Fam Behav Ther 1997;19(3):13–28.
30. McNeil C, Eyberg S, Eisenstadt T, et al. Parent-child interaction therapy with behavior problem children: generalization of treatment effects to the school setting. J Clin Child Psychol 1991;20:140–51.
31. McCabe KM, Yeh M, Garland AF, et al. The GANA program: a tailoring approach to adapting parent child interaction therapy for Mexican Americans. Education and Treatment of Children 2005;28(2):111–29.
32. Timmer SG, Urquiza AJ, Zebell NM. Challenging foster caregiver-maltreated child relationships: the effectiveness of parent-child interaction therapy. Child Youth Serv Rev 2006;28(1):1–19.
33. McNeil CB, Herschell AD, Gurwitch RH, et al. Training foster parents in parent-child interaction therapy. Education and Treatment of Children 2005;28:182–96.
34. Kolko DJ. Individual cognitive behavioral treatment and family therapy for physically abused children and their offending parents: a comparison of clinical outcomes. Child Maltreat 1996;1(4):322–42.
35. Cohen JA, Mannarino AP. A treatment model for sexually abused preschool children. J Interpers Violence 1993;8(1):115–31.
36. Deblinger E, Heflin AH. Treating sexually abused children and their nonoffending parents: a cognitive behavioral approach. Thousand Oaks, CA: Sage Publications; 1996.

37. Cohen JA, Deblinger E, Mannarino AP, et al. A multisite, randomized controlled trial for children with sexual abuse-related PTSD symptoms. J Am Acad Child Adolesc Psychiatry 2004;43(4):393–402.

38. Cohen JA, Mannarino AP, Knudsen K. Treating sexually abused children: one year follow-up of a randomized controlled trial. Child Abuse and Neglect 2005; 29(2):135–45.

39. Deblinger E, Steer RA, Lippmann J. Two year follow-up study of cognitive behavioral therapy for sexually abused children suffering posttraumatic stress symptoms. Child Abuse and Neglect 1999;23(12):1371–8.

40. Deblinger E, Mannarino AP, Cohen JA, et al. A follow-up study of a multisite, randomized controlled trial for children with sexual abuse-related PTSD symptoms. J Am Acad Child Adolesc Psychiatry 2006;45(12):1474–84.

41. Lieberman AF, Van Horn P. "Don't hit my mommy!": a manual for child-parent psychotherapy with young witnesses of family violence. Washington, DC: Zero to Three Press; 2005.

42. Cicchetti D, Rogosch FA, Toth SL. Fostering secure attachment in infants in maltreating families through preventive interventions. Dev Psychopathol 2006;18(3): 623–49.

43. Toth SL, Maughan A, Manly JT, et al. The relative efficacy of two interventions in altering maltreated preschool children's representational models: implications for attachment theory. Dev Psychopathol 2002;14(4):877–908.

44. Lieberman AF, Van Horn P, Ghosh Ippen C. Toward evidence-based treatment: child-parent psychotherapy with preschoolers exposed to marital violence. J Am Acad Child Adolesc Psychiatry 2005;44(12):1241–8.

45. Lieberman AF, Ghosh Ippen C, Van Horn P. Child-parent psychotherapy: 6-month follow-up of a randomized controlled trial. J Am Acad Child Adolesc Psychiatry 2006;45(8):913–8.

46. Cicchetti D, Toth SL, Rogosh FA. The efficacy of toddler-parent psychotherapy to increaseattachment security in offspring of depressed mothers. Attach Hum Dev 1999;1(1):34–66.

47. Lieberman AF, Weston DR, Pawl JH. Preventive intervention and outcomes with anxiously attached dyads. Child Dev 1991;62(1):199–209.

48. Taussig HN, Clyman RB, Landsverk J. Children who return home from foster care: a six-year prospective study of behavioral health outcomes in adolescence. Pediatrics 2001;108(1). Available at: http://www.pediatrics.org/cgi/content/full/108/1/ e10. Accessed October 28, 2008.

49. Taussig HN, Culhane SE. Foster care as an intervention for abused and neglected children. In: Kendall-Tackett KA, Giacomoni SM, editors. Child victimization: maltreatment, bullying and violence, prevention and intervention. Kingston, NJ: Civic Research Institute; 2005. p. 20: 1–20:25.

50. Barth RP. On their own: the experiences of youth after foster care. Child Adolesc Social Work J 1990;7(5):419–40.

51. Chapman MV, Wall A, Barth RP, et al. Children's voices: the perceptions of children in foster care. Am J Orthop 2004;74(3):293–304.

52. Courtney ME, Piliavin I, Grogan-Kaylor A. The Wisconsin study of youth aging out of out of home care: a portrait of children about to leave care. Madison, WI: School of Social Work, University of Wisconsin-Madison; 1995.

53. Johnson PR, Yoken C, Voss R. Family foster care placement: the child's perspective. Child Welfare 1995;74(5):960–74.

54. Nollan, KA, Arthur M, Pecora, PJ, et al. Relationships between risk factors and outcomes among youth in long-term foster care. Poster presented at the Biennial

Meetings of the Society for Research in Child Development. Albuquerque, NM, April 15–19, 1999.

55. Chamberlain P, Price J, Leve LD, et al. Prevention of behavior problems for children in foster care: outcomes and mediation effects. Prev Sci 2008;9(17):17–27.

56. Fisher PA, Gunnar MR, Chamberlain P, et al. Preventive intervention for maltreated preschool children: impact on children's behavior, neuroendocrine activity, and foster parent functioning. J Am Acad Child Adolesc Psychiatry 2000;39(11):1356–64.

57. Fisher PA, Burraston B, Pears K. The early intervention foster care program: permanent placement outcomes from a randomized trial. Child Maltreat 2005; 10(1):61–71.

58. Dozier M, Peloso E, Lindheim O, et al. Developing evidence-based interventions for foster children: an example of a randomized clinical trial with infants and toddlers. J Soc Issues 2006;62(4):767–85.

59. Linares OL, Montalto D, Li M, et al. A promising parenting intervention in foster care. J Consult Clin Psychol 2006;74(1):32–41.

60. Clark HB, Prange ME, Lee B, et al. Improving adjustment outcomes for foster children with emotional and behavioral disorders: early findings from a controlled study on individualized services. J Emot Behav Disord 1994;2(4):207–18.

61. Taussig HN, Culhane SE, Hettleman D. Fostering healthy futures: an innovative preventive intervention for preadolescent youth in out-of-home care. Child Welfare 2007;86(5):113–31.

62. Lutzker JR, Bigelow KM. Reducing child maltreatment: a guidebook for parent services. New York, NY: Guilford Publications; 2002.

Child Maltreatment Law and Policy as a Foundation for Child Advocacy

Donald C. Bross, JD, PhD[a],*, Richard D. Krugman, MD[b]

KEYWORDS

- Advocacy • Bioethics • Child abuse • Child neglect
- Rights of children • Policy • Pediatric law

The concept that child advocacy is a core pediatric task is advancing into the current century. The past 50 years of recognition and response to the battered child syndrome provide dramatic proof of the importance of pediatric advocacy. This experience illustrates the powerful effects of policy efforts by pediatricians and society at large to improve the lives of children. Pediatricians' success in aiding in the recognition and treatment of child abuse and neglect argues for systematic and sustained efforts to understand how pediatricians can advocate most effectively for children in all aspects of their health and development. Looking ahead, pediatricians should promote dedicated research on how advocacy for children is necessarily different from advocacy for other human interests and also, whatever the difficulties, how advocacy for children can best be advanced. Who better than pediatricians to bring all the tools of science, intergenerational professionalism, multidisciplinary partnerships, and visionary perspectives to advocacy for children?

It now is recognized that child abuse is an egregious and widespread problem. During 2 centuries of broad efforts, advocacy for children has helped improve children's education, prevent exploitation by way of child labor, and improve children's well being in other ways, such as safe milk and good diet. Specific activities by pediatricians included the diagnosis of the battered child and other conditions associated with maltreatment and the promotion of reporting laws and pilot programs to treat and prevent child abuse, which led to extensive and enduring changes in child welfare

This work was supported by the Kempe Foundation for the Prevention and Treatment of Child Abuse and Neglect.

[a] The Kempe Center for the Prevention and Treatment of Child Abuse and Neglect, University of Colorado School of Medicine, 13123 E. 16th Avenue, Box 390, Aurora, CO 80045, USA
[b] University of Colorado School of Medicine, 13001 E. 17th Place, Campus Box C290, Aurora, CO 80045, USA
* Corresponding author.
E-mail address: bross.doanld@tchden.org (D.C. Bross).

Pediatr Clin N Am 56 (2009) 429–439
doi:10.1016/j.pcl.2009.01.001
0031-3955/09/$ – see front matter © 2009 Elsevier Inc. All rights reserved.

pediatric.theclinics.com

systems and raised public awareness of the plight of deprived children. As new infor-mation about children's needs is developed, child advocacy can be improved substan-tially through the systematic study of when and how advocacy succeeds or fails.

THE INCIDENCE, PREVALENCE, AND COSTS OF CHILD MALTREATMENT

Modern attention to child abuse first arose through a series of improvements in diag-nosing the problem, beginning with recognition of the battered child syndrome.[1] Improvements in diagnosing many forms of physical child abuse were followed by more accurate diagnosis of nonorganic factors in failure to thrive, and this recognition was followed by improved diagnosis of sexual child abuse and other, rarer forms of maltreatment. The efforts of pediatricians and other health providers have led to a clearer understanding of how child maltreatment can cause immediate death or severe disability. Nationally, there are more than 800,000 confirmed reports of maltreatment every year, and the estimated number of yearly deaths exceeds 1000. Figures are more complete in the United States than in most countries because of mandatory reporting laws pioneered by pediatricians in the 1960s.[2] The experience in the United States has continued long enough to produce fairly stable year-to-year figures, and some apparent decreases in actual incidence have been seen.[3] The immediate health care costs of child abuse are illustrated by a health economist's study that found inflicted head injuries in infants predicted significantly greater (60% or more) costs and length of hospital stays than for children who suffered noninflicted head injuries.[4] As discussed later in this article, pediatricians have helped identify prevention and treatment programs that address child maltreatment.

Any form of child maltreatment, abuse, or neglect creates risk for short- and long-term harmful consequences such as physical and mental illness, including substance abuse[5] and criminality.[6] Risks to abused and neglected children have been deter-mined by many different methods. For example, in terms of crime prevention, retro-spective-prospective studies by Widom[7] seem to demonstrate that the risk for delinquent and criminal behavior later in life is about 60% greater for children identified by human services as having experienced maltreatment or victimization than for other children from the same environment. Prospective, random field trials conducted by Olds and colleagues[8] demonstrated that effective preventive nursing visitation for first-time mothers in need of extra services reduces child abuse, hospitalizations, direct costs for community services, and later criminal behavior. Additional studies conducted using various methods continue to show the range of social and economic costs of what now is proven to be an endemic societal problem afflicting many chil-dren and families.

BROADER "CHILD WELFARE" POLICY IN THE PAST 200 YEARS

To appreciate more accurately the influence of medical attention to child maltreat-ment, it should be remembered that such efforts are part of a broad tradition of child welfare advocacy and that that child welfare advocacy has played a central role within the broader context of child advocacy. Placing the influence of policy on the lives of children in a broader context shows that modern attention to specific injuries to chil-dren is the latest of a series of innovations on behalf of children that have been recog-nized as needed, have been implemented, and sometimes have been forgotten.

An important area of improvement in child well being is education. The Boston Latin School, founded April 23, 1635 by the Town of Boston, seems to be the first continu-ously open public school in the United States. The changing prevalence of public schools in the United States over the ensuing centuries is more difficult to document.

Nor is it easy to prove possible the effects of widely available public and sectarian schools on literacy. For a particular moment in time, however, we have a snapshot of the association between schools and literacy and the national economy. At the time of the Crystal Palace World's Fair in 1851, English businessmen attempted to understand the rapid rise of industry in the United States, which was remarkable even in comparison with the peaking Industrial Revolution in England. Embarking for the United States to discover factors in this rise, the English investigators found that by the 1850s more than 90% of the free population in the United States was literate, and in the New England states the literacy rate was 95%, compared with a literacy rate of about 65% in England.[9] Federal support for land grant colleges during the Civil War, the use of public education to help acculturate immigrants and improve social cohesion, and work on the importance of investment in "human capital" that won the Nobel Prize in economics[10] are all markers for the many ways in which American children's well being has been tied to larger human concerns.

Kindergartens began in Europe in the 1800s, were adopted in the United States by mid-century, and are found in many countries across the world. In Europe and the United States there have been numerous reforms in the management of orphanages and in the juvenile justice system. In Europe, for example, Janus Korczak did a great deal with progressive orphanages and involvement in juvenile justice.[11] After emigrating to the United States, psychiatrist Rene Spitz elaborated on the pioneering recognition of "hospitalism" by emphasizing the crucial importance of maternal care.[12] In the twentieth century, juvenile courts became common in Chicago, Denver, and other cities in the United States.

The issue of child labor also was addressed repeatedly, beginning in the Industrial Revolution. One of the early "Factory Acts" in England restricted the employment of children under the age of 12 in mines and factories. Remnants of this law are visible today: the Constitution of Colorado, for example, provides that "The general assembly … shall prohibit the employment in the mines of children under twelve years of age."[13] Between 1909 and 1912 the US Congress addressed child labor by creating the Children's Bureau, but as late as 1918 the US Supreme Court struck down certain elements of the law as an unconstitutional deprivation of a parent's rights to the fruits of a child's labor.[14]

Efforts to Benefit Children's Health Directly

As many pediatricians are aware, "taking a position on child health" was the catalyst for the founding of the American Academy of Pediatrics. In his tribute to Abraham Jacobi, Edmund Burke[15] wrote:

> [T]he Shepherd-Towner Act, which had been signed into law in 1921 and which was intended to be phased out in 1927, represented the first time that a federal grant program had been established in the field of health. This was a maternal and child health program. Despite the noble intent of this action by Congress, there was hue and cry against it by organized medicine.
>
> The dissatisfaction in the ranks of pediatrics members of the AMA persisted until finally in 1930, 35 pediatricians met in the Harper Hospital in Detroit, drew up a constitution and bylaws, and established a new society named the American Academy of Pediatrics. In the years that followed the pediatricians have attended the AMA meetings as a Section Council, with a delegate and alternate delegate, although at many times reluctantly or even dispiritedly. In earlier years, it must be admitted, the hearts of AAP [American Academy of Pediatrics] delegates were not into serving this role, because of the lack of satisfaction with AMA policies.

In the following decade the Shepherd-Towner Act was succeeded by the Social Security Act, unquestionably one of the most important child welfare efforts of the twentieth century. The Social Security Act, as amended, remains essential today as a national and local safety net in several areas of child well being. Benefited children include those whose parents are disadvantaged in various ways, including children who are orphaned or in foster care, have developmental disabilities, need preventive health services, or otherwise benefit directly and indirectly from Medicaid and Supplemental Security Income.

Pediatricians have been crucial in many efforts to address infectious disease in children, including leadership in small pox eradication,[16] polio vaccination, and national campaigns to assure high levels of childhood immunizations. Early periodic screening and diagnostic testing have proven effective in identifying and helping assure early treatment for many types of disability. As demonstrated by current decreases in immunization rates, even highly scientific programs to benefit children's health may not be sustained without continuing advocacy.

Noninflicted Injury

Pediatricians have been prominent in protecting children from two forms of trauma, non-inflicted and inflicted. Because non-inflicted trauma ("accidental injury") is a leading cause of death for children age 1 year and older in the United States,[17] pediatric advocacy is important and has proven successful in efforts to reduce poisoning, to lessen injuries from unsafe toys, and to mandate the use of car seats and seat belts. Research conducted by Kitzman and colleagues[18] in Memphis indicates that nursing visitation in early life can prevent many different injuries in early childhood, both noninflicted and inflicted.

Neglect can create immediate harm (eg, when children are not supervised near water or traffic or do not receive free or inexpensive immunizations). Neglect also leads to incremental harm. When there is a lack of active care, stimulation, mentoring, and anticipatory guidance throughout childhood, younger children can suffer from failure to grow physically (sometimes to the extent to psychosocial dwarfism) or can suffer other disabilities. Neglect can lead to poor socialization, emotional regulation, and poor academic achievement. Neglect is equivalent to physical abuse in its association with later outcomes of delinquency, crime,[19] and "futility syndrome" or intergenerationally transmitted hopelessness and helplessness.[20]

Inflicted Injury

Mandatory reporting of suspected child abuse followed 11 years after the published description of the battered child syndrome.[1] Even today only a few countries mandate reporting of child abuse or neglect;[21] in most countries, the reporting of child abuse is not legally required, and child abuse is vastly underreported.[22] Even in countries that nominally encourage reporting as a professional and ethical responsibility, the lack of protections for reporters, found in United States law, seems to discourage the recognition and response to the problem in much of the world.

In addressing child fatalities, short- and long-term disability, and the creation of risk for long-term physical, behavioral, and social harms from maltreatment, the discussion immediately becomes complicated by the need for institutional and societal responses. Solutions necessary for some children, such as foster care, can become points of contention well before scientific studies can clarify how to decide when foster care must be avoided and how to assure that, if placement is necessary, the experience for the child and family is made as beneficial as possible. Similarly, studies on the effects of various approaches to family treatment have been conducted only in the past few decades, especially during the past 10 years, but policies on intervention have changed repeatedly, based on sensational stories and the perception that corrections in the existing system were necessary. When essentially nonscientific institutions, such as the courts, are involved, research on the positive and negative effects of their intervention has been even slower to appear. In response to various challenges to previous practice, qualified researchers and funding agencies finally are giving more attention to inflicted injury. Without the impetus from pediatricians to implement the recommendations of scientifically based literature on preventing child abuse, there would be less likelihood of evidenced-based practices related to child maltreatment, slowing the rate of progress in this area (and in many other conditions related to children's health).

PEDIATRICS AS A FOUNDATION FOR POLICY AND LAW RELATED TO CHILDHOOD

A specific example of pediatricians' direct involvement in advocacy is the role pediatricians have played in providing testimony in court cases involving children. Pediatric testimony in court about child maltreatment can be essential in many child protection proceedings, some contested divorces, and even in a few juvenile justice cases. In such cases the pediatrician is not the legal advocate for the child but instead provides evidenced-based information about a child's condition and needs. In effect, the pediatrician provides the facts that can speak for children too young or impaired to speak for themselves.[23] Accountability for preventable child fatalities often occurs only through pediatric testimony.[24] More broadly, Dr. Barton Schmitt provided essential testimony in the landmark case of *Landeros v. Flood*,[25] which established the judicial precedent for professional responsibility for failure to report suspected child abuse. Desmond Runyan[26] helped pioneer research showing that most abused children who are old enough to testify can manage the experience and that, for those who can testify, there are interventions that make it more likely that any trauma experienced will be transitory.

These examples serve only to introduce and illustrate the ways pediatric knowledge can change law, public opinion, and policy with respect to childhood well being. Pediatricians' development of a medical focus on the unique health needs of children has led broadly to important improvements in professional care for children. Pediatricians have fostered an appreciation of the importance of childhood experiences for later life and the power of early intervention to reshape subsequent life spans, productivity, and overall costs for society. Pediatricians have succeeded in creating pediatric principles of practice that range from helping people understand why a child is not a "little adult," to promoting scientific innovations such as microchemistry, to responding as allies to the needs of parents eager to give their children the best possible care. Pediatricians have been especially helpful to parents in need of support for their parenting. Pediatricians simultaneously have helped elevate the status of childhood at a time when of many types investments in childhood can be shown to yield enormous returns. It is surprising, therefore, that pediatricians as a whole have not always promoted specific research to advance the science and the profession of child advocacy as an academic subspecialty, either as an allied profession or as a specific, science-based activity within pediatrics.

Evidence-based practice in pediatrics usually emphasizes the importance of science. New practices can be established as safe and efficacious, and old practices can be challenged as unwise or even harmful. Thus, pediatrics has built-in accountability for the practices and positions of the profession to a degree that most other child-caring professions do not. Many other professions devoted to the improvement of children's lives also rely on science, but no other professional body seems to accept and endorse such a wide variety of inquiries into the complex lives of children. Pediatricians both engage in and use evidence-based biologic science and behavioral science.

In seeking a general framework for pediatric principles, practice, and policy, perhaps the most comprehensive health framework for fruitfully combining medical and behavioral research, law, politics, and policy to advocate for children is a public health model. Within public health institutions and traditions, all public and private, primary, secondary, and tertiary prevention or treatment services can be encompassed. Fifty years ago, no single preventive strategy (other than addressing poverty through income supplements) had been identified that would reduce poverty, unwanted pregnancy, substance abuse, delinquency and crime, and hospitalization. In the 1970s Henry Kempe and his colleagues tried to prevent severe physical abuse of children by using paraprofessional home visitors, and their pilot program did succeed.[27] Psychologist David Olds expanded the research theory and improved the initial outcome by using nurses with a much richer theoretical and practical protocol, demonstrating that all these outcomes could be achieved in select populations.[8] Currently, psychologist Gary Melton is trying a broader community-based approach to social and mental health "community immunization" as another way of dealing with "vectors of harm" that endanger children and of delivering services to underserved populations.[28] Underlying these efforts is the original breakthrough revealed by pediatric research documenting the extent and direct implications of severe trauma within families.

Advocacy has been an integral part of the development of pediatrics as a profession. One of the highest honors that can be bestowed on an American pediatrician is the Jacobi Award. To understand the importance of this award in the pediatric tradition, one can to return to Edmund Burke's[15] biography of Abraham Jacobi published in *Pediatrics* in 1998. After enumerating Jacobi's extraordinary accomplishments, Burke concluded that, most of all, Jacobi represents the fundamental and crucial role that pediatricians play in advocacy.

> *I view the legacy of Abraham Jacobi as advocacy. Advocacy in pediatrics is the name of the game. Jacobi showed us the way, but others have followed suit in such an effective campaign that today we have the AAP [American Academy of Pediatrics] representing nearly 60 000 pediatricians eminent in the nation as well as in the halls of Congress in the advocacy role.*

Most pediatricians probably would agree with the concept that advocacy is a core value of pediatrics. The range of what has been accomplished and what remains to be done in a systematic fashion should encourage all pediatricians to advocate whenever possible and appropriate.

Forms of Advocacy

Advocacy means different things to different people. One of the purposes of this article is to demonstrate the range of methods that can be used to advocate for children's well being, the levels at which advocacy for children can occur, and the need for research to investigate more systematically how to use most effectively whatever method may be employed. The following range of activities begins to frame the challenge and potential of pediatric advocacy as a study in itself.

Professional identity and membership

The American Academy of Pediatrics and comparable pediatrics-focused membership organizations have been instrumental in advocating for children in many of the most important areas of health reform and improvement. As evidence of the extent of the advocacy efforts of the American Academy of Pediatrics, there are 91 awards for achievements within the pediatric tradition. Many of these awards recognize not science or teaching but a specific type of pediatric advocacy by name. These awards tap into individual professional interests and competencies and also demonstrate the great range of advocacy activities that are useful, from local to national, and from very specific to broad-stroke approaches.

Legislation locally
Legislative advocacy has been an important avenue for improvements in children's health since the beginning of pediatrics as a field. With time, pediatricians are learning more effective and practical ways to advocate in the legislative arena[29] and are realizing that pediatricians can be trained specifically to be effective advocates.[30]

Individual, family, and anticipatory guidance with individual patients
Partnerships with parents are a crucial form of pediatric advocacy in which pediatricians and parents together monitor the growth and development, problems, and proper response to the enormous variety of illnesses, developmental delays, traumas, and challenges that every child encounters to a greater or lesser degree.

Public education and working with the media
Parents and pediatricians should not be alone in supporting programs for the benefit of children. Many examples can be cited of the importance of public education in advocacy and policy work for children, including current efforts to reduce smoking, especially by young people. Advertising campaigns funded by the Chicago-based National Center for the Prevention of Child Abuse (now Prevent Child Abuse America) in the 1970s were intended to promote the reporting of suspected child abuse. The Ad Council was a co-sponsor, and a number of private and public corporations supported the public education campaign. Eventually, the group moved to prevention through paraprofessional home visitation, attempting to implement through state legislation Ray Helfer's idea of "Children's Trust Funds" as a source for needed prevention funding. At certain times in the campaign to encourage reporting, the ability of state systems to respond adequately was overwhelmed. Thus the campaign was both a success and an example of the need for better science-based policy as part of public education campaigns.

At any one moment, the media can both clarify and confuse the understanding of crucial health issues involving children. Timely and carefully crafted interviews and editorials are an important form of pediatric advocacy.[31]

Academic and private foundation programs
The power of investments in foundational intellectual approaches to policy is demonstrated by the recent history of conservative and liberal politics in the United States. In an analogous way, there is a natural need to relate children's healthy development to politics, economics, law, and bioethics. As one example, there is an inherent inverse association between an emphasis on beneficence versus an emphasis on autonomy; autonomy is related directly to competency, and competency in turn is related to maturation. For example, research has demonstrated that adolescents charged with an offense often are not competent to advise legal counsel.[32] Needed are a considered ethical basis for thinking about childhood and a policy that recognizes that "substituted judgment" is more difficult for individuals who have not lived very long

and that it is easier to misconstrue what these individually really might want to be done for them were they somehow able to consider maturely the implications of available options. Bioethics devoted to childhood is a necessary focus if the power of modern medicine is to be managed in a way that assures adherence to the principle of "first do no harm." Pediatric law and bioethics must develop to help pediatricians and other child advocates understand more clearly what should be done.

Pediatrics must encourage the development of a subspecialty of law, ideally pairing it with pediatric bioethics, to help articulate meaningful and enforceable rights of children, beginning with clarity about the legal interests of children, both together with and apart from other members of society. Included are questions of when a child is sufficiently mature to make certain decisions, how best to understand the legal authority of parents over children and the claims of children on their parents, how to distinguish better between the nonparental claims of any number of adults and their organizations, what standards of care should be imposed for different caregivers of children, and what safeguards are necessary to assure accountability when adults purport to speak on behalf of children. Pediatric law must develop to help advocates understand what must be done, and pediatric bioethics must elucidate what should be done.

The ideal enterprise for establishing this work would embed all aspects of the law, the bioethics of child development, and the science of pediatric medical care within an academic program of pediatric law and pediatric bioethics. Because law, courts, and law schools have proven that they do not yet provide an environment in which they can focus every day on the "business of childhood" from the bottom up, rather than applying adult analogues to the lives of children from the top down, it seems that only in advanced pediatrics and children's hospital settings can this work be incubated well enough to foster what is required.

Research is needed on the forms that advocacy for children can take and the ways different forms of advocacy can be made effective. A few of areas needing further study are outlined here.

Courtroom and appellate legal advocacy

C. Henry Kempe managed the establishment of International Society for the Prevention and Treatment of Child Abuse and Neglect and its associated publication, *Child Abuse and Neglect*, in 1977, and thereby helped established a sound scientific basis for advocacy for children. Kempe simultaneously endorsed the establishment of the National Association of Counsel for Children (NACC). Kempe recognized that although competent pediatric expert testimony could make a great difference for abused children, the competency of the attorney representing the child also could make a crucial difference in how well the testimony was presented and how thoroughly the child's legal interests were addressed. As always, Kempe was "team oriented" and saw how many different professions need to collaborate to achieve the best possible results. The NACC, which has more than 2500 members, trains lawyers for children to be competent in court, trains pediatric and child psychiatry witnesses to be good witnesses, tests and accredits Child Welfare Law Specialists under the aegis of the American Bar Association, and files *amicus curiae* in state courts of last resort and the Federal courts on issues of "general importance to children." The current President of the NACC is a pediatrician, demonstrating the benefits for children gained from the mutual support and interaction between pediatricians and lawyers for children.

Opportunities exist for pediatricians to help educate judges about children's issues when they arrive in the courts. Despite the large number of "family court" cases heard in local courts and on appeal, a very small percentage of *amicus curiae* briefs are filed in appellate cases involving the lives of children, especially as compared with other legal appeals. Children's lives, especially lives in caught in conflict or excessive risk, could be improved by making better knowledge available to decision makers.[33,34]

State, federal, and international legislation

Much, and perhaps most, legislation takes a "top down" approach to implementing change. United States Public Law 93-247, for example, provided small amounts of additional Federal funding for states that adopted consistent elements in their reporting laws. This funding helped make reporting laws in the United States more uniform, with important features such as protection against liability for good faith reporting by physicians and others. The encouragement of reporting, however, was not supported consistently by other Federal efforts to assure that state child welfare systems can meet the task of responding appropriately to such reports. In understanding and applying different strategies and tactics for advocacy, one must recognize that each approach can have advantages and disadvantages. Another useful example of such tradeoffs is the United Nations Convention on the Rights of the Child. Aside from the Sudan, the United States seems to be the lone nonsignatory in the world community. The United States could do what many countries have done: ratify the Convention for the sake of expediency, formally taking as many "exceptions" as needed to limit its impact on American tradition and law (both common law and Constitutional law). Among the aspects of the United Nations Convention likely to result in conflict (and even in Constitutional challenges in the United States.) are provisions that children have rights before birth, that the state must assure that the "best interests" of children are observed, and that there can be no discrimination based on race, religion, or several other attributes. The potential of the first example for exciting political conflict obvious. Currently, the "best interest" standard cannot be used as a justification for state intervention in the lives of children who might be maltreated; the state is permitted (and, indeed, required) to act in the child's best interests only after it is more likely than not that a child has been abused (or when the child is dependent on the state). The Indian Child Welfare Act clearly "discriminates" against Native American children as individuals because it requires that maltreatment of these children, unlike most children in the United States, must be proven by "clear and convincing" evidence. A child can be freed for adoption because of abuse only if the evidence is proven beyond a reasonable doubt. This differential treatment, however, has been justified as a means of maintaining tribal integrity in the face of documented discrimination. In many areas, such as child labor, use of children in the military, public education, and health care, children are very much better off in the United States than in some of the countries that have ratified the Convention. These countries observe the Convention in the breech rather than in reality. In the words of Chicago law professor Jack Goldsmith, "Here is something that critics of the [American] double standard tend to ignore: international human rights law inevitably involves a trade-off between ambition and legitimacy."

SUMMARY

Without sustained pediatric advocacy, many advances in children's health will not be sustained. Evidence-based policy supported by research, stories of success, case-by-case advocacy, pediatric "policy science," and the development of allied careers, especially in pediatric law and bioethics, are all needed to advance child advocacy. Pediatricians must support research that determines effective strategies for advocacy for a population that does not have the advantages adults enjoy have in advocating for themselves but might have other advantages, if these can be identified and implemented. The traditions and successes of pediatric advocacy, illustrated by pediatricians' work on behalf of abused and neglected children, are dramatic proof that pediatricians' advocacy is necessary for advances in children's health. Advocacy by individual pediatricians and by the profession as a whole should be evidence based and advanced by a degree of specialization and the establishment of allied professional careers in pediatric law and bioethics.

REFERENCES

1. Kempe CH, Silverman FN, Steele BF, et al. The battered child syndrome. JAMA 1962;181:17–24.
2. Paulsen MG. Child abuse reporting laws: the shape of the legislation. Columbia Law Rev 1967;67(1):1–36.
3. Finkelhor D, Jones L. Why have child maltreatment and child victimization declined? J Soc Issues 2006;62(4):685–716.
4. Libby AM, Marion R, Sills R, et al. Costs of childhood physical abuse: comparing inflicted and unintentional traumatic brain injuries. Pediatrics 2003;112(1):58–65.
5. Moeller TP, Bachmann GA, Moeller JR. The combined effects of physical, sexual, and emotional abuse during childhood: long-term health consequences for women. Child Abuse Negl 1993;17:623–40.
6. Lewis DO, Shavok SS, Pineus JH, et al. Violent juvenile delinquents: psychiatric, neurological, psychological, and abuse factors. J Am Acad Child Psychiatry 1979;18:307–17.
7. Widom CS, Maxfield MG. A prospective examination of risk for violence among abused and neglected children. In: Ferris C, Grisso T, editors. Understanding aggressive behavior in children, Ann N Y Acad Sci; 1994(794). p. 224–37.
8. Olds DL, Eckenrode J, Henderson CR, et al. Long-term effects of home visitation on maternal life course and child abuse and neglect: 15-year follow-up of a randomized trial. JAMA 1997;278(8):637–43.
9. Ehrlick E, Garland SB. Needed: human capital. Bus Week 1988;100–36.
10. Marshall E. Nobel prize for theory of economic growth. Science 1987;138:754–5.
11. Lifton BJ. The king of children: the life and death of Janusz Korczak. New York: St. Martins Griffin, ISBN 0-312-15560-3; 1988.
12. Crandall FM. Editorial. Arch Pediatr 1897;14(6):448–54.
13. Constitution of Colorado. Article XVI, Mining and Irrigation. Section 2.
14. Hammer v. Dagenhart, 247 U.S. 251, 1918.
15. Burke EC. Abraham Jacobi MD. The man and his legacy. Pediatrics 1998;10(2):309–12.
16. Kempe CH. The end of routine smallpox vaccination. Am J Dis Child 1972;49:489.
17. National Center for Health Statistics. Available at: http://209.217.72.34/HDAA/TableViewer/tableView.aspx?ReportId=274. Accessed August 26, 2008.
18. Kitzman H, Olds DL, Henderson CR Jr, et al. Effect of prenatal and infant home visitation by nurses on pregnancy outcomes, childhood injuries, and repeated childbearing: a randomized controlled trial. JAMA 1997;278(8):644–52.
19. Olds D, Henderson CR, Cole R. Long-term effects of home visitation on children's criminal and antisocial behavior: 15 year follow-up of a randomized controlled trial. JAMA 1998;280(14):1238–44.
20. Polansky NA, Williams DP, Buttenweiser EW. Damaged parents. Chicago: University of Chicago Press; 1983.

21. Bross DC, Miyoshi PK, Krugman RD. World perspectives on child abuse (The Fifth International Resource Book). Denver (CO): The International Society for the Prevention of Child Abuse and Neglect (ISPCAN) and the Kempe Children's Center, University of Colorado School of Medicine; 2002.
22. Mathews B, Bross DC. Mandated reporting is still a policy with reason: empirical evidence and philosophical grounds. Child Abuse Negl 2008;32(5):511–6.
23. Estele v. McGuire, 112 Sup. Ct. 475 (1991).
24. Krugman RD. Fatal child abuse: analysis of 24 cases. Pediatrician 1985;12: 68–72.
25. 17 Cal. 3d 399, 551 P.2d 389, 131 Cal. Rptr. 69 (Cal. 1976).
26. Runyan DK. The emotional impact of societal intervention into child abuse. In: Goodman GS, Bottoms BI, editors. Child victims and child witnesses: understanding and improving testimony. New York: Guilford; 1993. p. 263–77.
27. Gray J, Cutler C, Dean J, et al. Prediction and prevention of child abuse and neglect. J Soc Issues 1979;35(2):127–39.
28. Strong communities as safe havens for children. Fam Community Health 2008; 31(2).
29. Berman S. Getting it right for children: stories of pediatric care and advocacy. Elk Grove Village, IL: American Academy of Pediatrics; 2007.
30. Berman S. Training pediatricians to become child advocates. Pediatrics 1998; 102(3):632–5.
31. Krugman RD. The media and public awareness of child abuse and neglect: it's time for a change. Child Abuse Negl 1996;20(4):259–60.
32. Griss T, Steinberg L, Woolard J, et al. Juveniles' competence to stand trial: a comparison of adolescents' and adults' capacities as trial defendants. Law Hum Behav 2005;27(4):333–63.
33. Corbally SF, Bross DC, Flango EV. Filing of *amicus curiae* briefs in state courts of last resort 1960–2000. Justice System Journal 2004;25(1):39–56.
34. Flango EV, Corbally SF, Bross DC. *Amicus curiae*: the court's perspective. Justice System Journal 2006;27(2):180–90.

Index

Note: Page numbers of article titles are in **boldface** type.

A

Abuse. *See* Child abuse.
Abuse-Focused-Cognitive Behavioral Therapy, 419–421
Academic performance, in child neglect, 364
Advocacy, for child abuse and neglect prevention, 374, 399–400, **429–439**
    forms of, 434–436
    history of, 430–433
    legal, 436–437
    pediatrician involvement in, 433–437
    statistics relevant to, 430
Airway management, for head trauma, 325
Alcohol abuse. *See* Substance abuse.
Anticipatory guidance, for child abuse prevention, 435
Attachment and Biobehavioral Catch-up intervention, 423

B

Babygram, in head trauma, 324
Battered child syndrome. *See* Head trauma.
Bioethics, for child abuse prevention, 435–436
Bleeding disorders, versus abusive head trauma, 322
Bone scan, in head trauma, 324–325
Born to Learn curriculum, 395
Boston Latin School, 430–431
Brain trauma. *See* Head trauma.
Breastfeeding, substances of abuse transmitted in, 351
Burke, Edmund, on Jacobi advocacy for child welfare, 431–432, 434

C

Cameras, for retinal hemorrhage documentation, 337
Chemicals, accidental exposure to, 353–354
Child abuse
    costs of, 320
    epidemiology of, 320
    fatality in, 323, 326, 364, **379–387**
    head trauma in, **317–331**
    in foster are, **405–415**
    legal issues in, 379–380, **429–439**
    mental health treatment for, **417–428**
    neglect as. *See* Child neglect.

Pediatr Clin N Am 56 (2009) 441–448
doi:10.1016/S0031-3955(09)00026-1
0031-3955/09/$ – see front matter © 2009 Elsevier Inc. All rights reserved.

pediatric.theclinics.com

Child abuse (*continued*)
    prevention of, 326, **389–403**
    recidivism in, 396–397
    retinal hemorrhages in, 323, **333–344**
    substance abuse and. *See* Substance abuse.
Child neglect, **363–378**
    addressing, 372–373
    advocacy in, 374
    assessment of, 372
    chronicity of, 370
    cognitive effects of, 364
    context of, 370–371
    continuum of care and, 365–366
    costs of, 364
    definition of, 365–371
    environmental hazards and, 370
    epidemiology of, 363–364
    etiology of, 371–372
    evidence-based definition of, 366
    factors affecting, 370–371
    failure to thrive in, 369
    fatality in, 323, 326, 364
    frequency of, 370
    harm in, actual versus potential, 366–367
    health care issues in, 367–369
    heterogeneous nature of, 367–370
    importance of, 363–364
    in substance abuse, 351, 354
    intentionality of, 370
    moral issues in, 364
    morbidity in, 364
    new forms of, 370
    overweight in, 369
    parental responsibility and blame for, 365
    physical effects of, 364
    prevention of, 373–374
    rights of child and, 364–365
    severity of, 370
    substance abuse and, 369
Child protective services, for neglect cases, 363–378
Children's Trust Funds, 435
Chronicity, of child neglect, 370
Coagulation disorders, versus abusive head trauma, 322
Cocaine
    accidental ingestion of, 351–352
    fetal effects of, 349
Cognitive dysfunction, in child neglect, 364
Compliance, with health care recommendations, 367
Computed tomography, in head trauma, 324–325
Congenital malformations, versus abusive head trauma, 321
Context, of child neglect, 370–371

Council on Child and Adolescent Health, 393–394
Cultural attitudes, toward death in child abuse, 384

D

Death. *See* Fatality.
Drug abuse. *See* Substance abuse.

E

Early Intervention Foster Care program, 423
Early Intervention Program, 396
Edema, cerebral, 324, 338
Education, public, for child abuse prevention, 435
Elmira nurse-family partnership program, 391–393, 397–399
Environmental dangers
    of substance abuse, 350–354
    protection against, 370
Ethical issues, in child abuse, 435–436

F

Failure to thrive, 369
Falls, head trauma in, 322
Fatality, in child abuse and neglect, 364
    forensic considerations in, 323
    head trauma, 326
    review teams for, **379–387**
        case intake by, 382
        cultural attitudes and, 384
        follow-up by, 383
        growth of, 383–384
        history of, 379–382
        informal peer support for, 380
        membership of, 382
        new resources and challenges for, 383–384
        outcomes of, 384–385
        overview of, 379–380
        pediatrician involvement in, 385–386
        problems with, 383
        purpose of, 382
        structure of, 382
Fetal alcohol spectrum disorder, 348
Forensic considerations, in head trauma, 322–323
Foster care, **405–415**
    challenges in, 410
    health care needs in, 406
    mental health treatment for, 422–424
    needed reform in, 412–413
    placement instability in, 406–411
    statistics on, 405

Fostering Healthy Futures trial, 424
Fostering Success Act of 2008, 408–409
Foundations, for child abuse prevention, 435–436
Fractures
    long bone, in head trauma, 318, 323
    rib, 323, 337
    skull, 324–325
Frequency, of child neglect incidents, 370

G

Genetic disorders, versus abusive head trauma, 321–322
Genital injuries, with head trauma, 323
Glutaric aciduria, versus abusive head trauma, 322

H

Harm, actual versus potential, 366–367
Hawaii Health Start Program, 390, 394
Head trauma, **317–331**
    diagnosis of, 319–321
    differential diagnosis of, 321–322
    epidemiology of, 317–318
    forensic considerations in, 322–323
    imaging in, 324–325
    injuries associated with, 323–324
    mechanisms of, 318–319
    outcomes of, 325–326, 340–341
    prevention of, 326
    retinal hemorrhages in. *See* Retinal hemorrhages.
    spectrum of, 317
    terminology of, 317
    timing of, 325
    treatment of, 325
Health care, for children
    adequacy of, 365–366
    delay in receiving, 367–369
    in foster care, 405–415
    noncompliance with, 367
Healthy Families America, 394–395
Hearing loss, in head trauma, 326
Hematoma
    scalp, 318
    subdural, 318, 320–322, 325
Hemiplegia, in head trauma, 326
Hemorrhages, retinal. *See* Retinal hemorrhages.
Heroin, fetal effects of, 349
Home visiting programs, for child abuse prevention, **389–403**
    advocacy implications of, 399–400
    evolution of, 390–393

expansion of, 393–394
   primary care provider involvement in, 400
   public policy for, 399–400
   replication of programs, 398–399
   research on, 394–398
Hydrocephalus, in head trauma, 326

I

Incredible Years parenting program, 423
Indian Child Welfare Act, 437
Inflicted injuries
   head. *See* Head trauma.
   protection against, 432–433
Intentionality, of child neglect, 370
Interagency Council on Child Abuse and Neglect, fatality review by, 380
International Society for the Prevention and Treatment of Child Abuse and Neglect, 436
Intracranial hemorrhage, asymptomatic, 321
Intracranial pressure, increased, retinal hemorrhages in, 338
Intrathoracic pressure, increased, retinal hemorrhage in, 337–338

J

Jacobi, Abraham, as child welfare advocate, 431–432, 434

K

Kauffman Best Practices Project, 419
Keeping Foster Parents Trained and Supported trial, 422
Kempe, Henry, as child welfare advocate, 434, 436

L

Landeros v. Flood child abuse case, 433
Legal issues, in child abuse and neglect, **429–439**
   courtroom advocacy, 436–437
   early legislation, 379–380
   history of, 430–433
   legislation, 435, 437
   pediatrician involvement in, 433–437
   statistics relevant to, 430
Legislation, for child abuse prevention, 379–380, 435, 437

M

Magnetic resonance imaging, in head trauma, 324–325
Marijuana
   accidental ingestion of, 352
   fetal effects of, 348–349
Media connections, for child abuse prevention, 435
Medicaid, for foster children, 409

Melton, Gary, as child welfare advocate, 434

Menkes kinky hair disease, versus abusive head trauma, 322

Mental health treatment, in child abuse and neglect, **417–428**
    cognitive behavioral therapy for, 420–421
    evidence-based practices for, 418–424
    in foster care, 422–424
    parenting interventions for, 420–421
    psychotherapy for, 421–422
    statistics on, 417–418
    types of disorders and, 418

Metabolic disorders, versus abusive head trauma, 321–322

Methadone
    fetal effects of, 349
    parental administration of, 352–353

Methamphetamine
    accidental ingestion of, 352
    clandestine laboratories manufacturing, 353–355
    fetal effects of, 349–350
    passive exposure to, 353

Moral issues, in child neglect, 364

Multidimensional Treatment Foster Care program, 422

N

Narcotics, fetal effects of, 349

National Association of Counsel for Children, 436

National Center for the Prevention of Child Abuse, 435

National Child Traumatic Stress Network, 419–420

National Commission to Prevent Infant Mortality, 393–394

A Nation's Shame, Fatal Child Abuse and Neglect in the United States, 381–382

Neglect. *See* Child neglect.

Neonatal abstinence syndrome, 356

Nonaccidental head trauma. *See* Head trauma.

Noncompliance, with health care recommendations, 367

Non-inflicted injury, protection against, 432

Northwest Foster Care Alumni study, 406

Nurse(s), in home visiting programs. *See* Home visiting programs.

Nurse-family partnership program, 391–393, 397–399

O

Olds, David, as child welfare advocate, 434

Opioids, fetal effects of, 349

Optic nerve injury, 341

Osteogenesis imperfecta, versus abusive head trauma, 322

Overweigh children, 369

P

Papilledema, in head trauma, 338

Parent-Child Interaction Therapy, 419–420

Parents as Teachers program, 390–391, 394–396
Photodocumentation, of retinal hemorrhages, 337
Pregnancy, substance abuse in, 347–350
Prevent Child Abuse America, 394, 435
Project Safecare, 396–397
Psychosocial effects, of child neglect, 364
Psychotherapy, child-parent, 421–422
Psychotropic drugs, for children in foster care, 407–408
Purtscher syndrome, 337

Q

Quadriplegia, in head trauma, 326

R

Radiography, in head trauma, 324–325
Retinal hemorrhages, 323, **333–344**
    anatomic considerations in, 335
    animal models of, 339–340
    causes of, 323
    differential diagnosis of, 334
    documentation of, 333–337
    epidemiology of, 323–324, 333
    imaging in, 324
    locations of, 335–336
    mechanisms of, 337–339
    outcomes of, 340–341
Retinoschisis, in hemorrhage, 335–336, 340
"Reversal sign," in head trauma, 324
Rib fractures, 323, 337
Rights, of children, 364–365, 437

S

SafeCare Program, 424
Scalp, hematoma of, 318
Scintigraphy, in head trauma, 324–325
Second impact syndrome, 322
Seizures, in head trauma, 325
Severity, of child neglect, 370
Shaken infant syndrome. See Head trauma.
Shepherd-Towner Act, 431–432
Skeletal survey, in head trauma, 324
Skull radiography, in head trauma, 324–325
Sleep position, 370
Smoke, second-hand, 370
Socioeconomic factors, in head trauma, 320
Subdural hematoma, 318, 320–322, 325

Substance abuse
    child ingestion and, 351–353
    child maltreatment in, **345–362**
        environmental dangers and, 350–354
        epidemiology of, 345–346
        management of, 354–358
        prenatal, 347–350
        risk factors for, 346–347
    child neglect and, 369
    drug testing in, 355–356
    neonatal effects of, 369
    passive exposure to children, 353
    reporting of, 357–358
    treatment of, 356–357

T

Tardieu, Ambrose, as fatality review team pioneer, 379–380
Team approach
    to fatality review, **379–387**
    to head trauma diagnosis, 319
Terson syndrome, 338
Thrombophilia, retinal hemorrhage in, 339
Trauma
    head, **317–331**
    protection against, 432–433
Trauma-focused Cognitive Behavioral Therapy, 419

U

United Nations Convention on the Rights of the Child, 437

V

Veno-occlusive disease, retinal hemorrhage in, 339
Ventilation, for head trauma, 325
Visitation, home. See Home visiting programs.
Visual impairment
    in head trauma, 326
    in retinal hemorrhage, 340–341
Vitamin D deficiency, retinal hemorrhage in, 339
Vitreoretinal traction, hemorrhage in, 338–339

W

Whiplash injury. See Head trauma.
Wraparound services, for mental health issues, 423–424

Moving?

Make sure your subscription moves with you!

To notify us of your new address, find your **Clinics Account Number** (located on your mailing label above your name), and contact customer service at:

E-mail: elspcs@elsevier.com

800-654-2452 (subscribers in the U.S. & Canada)
314-453-7041 (subscribers outside of the U.S. & Canada)

Fax number: 314-523-5170

Elsevier Periodicals Customer Service
11830 Westline Industrial Drive
St. Louis, MO 63146

*To ensure uninterrupted delivery of your subscription, please notify us at least 4 weeks in advance of move.

Printed and bound by CPI Group (UK) Ltd, Croydon, CR0 4YY

03/10/2024

01040443-0016